The Life-Changing *Magic* of Quitting Alcohol

The Life-Changing Magic of *Magic* of Quitting Alcohol

Sharon Hartley

Aurum

Quarto

First published in 2025 by Aurum Press,
an imprint of The Quarto Group.
One Triptych Place, London, SE1 9SH,
United Kingdom
T (0)20 7700 9000
www.Quarto.com

EEA Representation, WTS Tax d.o.o., Žanova ulica 3, 4000 Kranj, Slovenia

A catalogue record for this book is available from the British Library.

ISBN 978-1-83600-152-2
Ebook ISBN 978-1-83600-153-9
Audiobook ISBN 978-1-83600-617-6

10 9 8 7 6 5 4 3 2 1

Typeset in Adobe Garamond Pro by seagulls.net
Printed by CPI group (UK) Ltd, Croydon, CR0 4YY

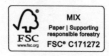

For Team Hartley,
Anna, Jeanette and Shani

CONTENTS

CHAPTER 1

• • • • • • • • • • •

What's so great about quitting alcohol?

How much time have you spent thinking about your relationship with alcohol? And how many hours do you reckon you have spent feeling hungover, or just a bit grouchy and sub-par, because you drank too much?

And how much time have you spent imagining how great life could be without any booze in it?

Well, that's what we're going to do here. This book is not a lecture on the perils of drinking designed to make you feel full of remorse whenever you so much as look at a glass of wine and regret all the times you had one (or several) too many. I promise you now that this is a shame-free zone.

Instead, it's a celebration of the joy that comes when you cut out the booze and focus on yourself: who you are and all the things you can achieve. When you ditch the alcohol and start living for you, instead of focusing on getting to that gin and tonic or cold beer at the end of the day that you tell yourself will make it all OK, Very Good Things can come your way.

In fact, I want to show you how stopping drinking can be one of the most rewarding things you can do for your future self.

Whether you are simply tired of your social life revolving around drinking, you would just like to kick a one-wine-a-night habit that you've realised slows you down the next day, or you are regularly writing off whole weekends due to being on a carousel of over-indulging and feeling horrendous, if you've picked up this book, changing your relationship with alcohol is probably something you've been debating in your head for a while. Maybe even years. However, when it comes to actually doing something concrete about it, you have likely found yourself floundering, going round in circles, making excuses, stalling and then putting it off until the 'right time' for fear of how a life without alcohol will look and even what other people might think.

I want this book to show you that no matter how much or how little you're drinking, a life without any alcohol in it is breathtakingly beautiful, exciting, full of opportunity and adventure, surprising, calm, colourful and utterly magical. Genuinely. I wouldn't have believed it myself had I not stopped drinking because once upon a time booze featured heavily in my life, and the idea of removing it entirely sounded utterly bonkers to me. Nonetheless, I stopped drinking and started properly living, and I want you to know this is possible for you too.

If alcohol is impacting your life negatively at whatever level, it's OK to acknowledge that. I don't care about your current units per week – I just want you to know that on the other side of boozing retirement is a life better than you ever thought possible. Of course, it's not without its challenges: there are moments when it can take balls of steel and it requires you to give it everything. As with just about anything in life, nothing will change if you tackle this half-arsed. You need to run at it with your full arse only. Only then will you begin to see change and reap the many, many benefits of a beautiful life no longer tainted or slightly stained by booze and its aftershocks. I want you to trust me when I wheel out this well-known line: 'The best views come after the hardest climb.' Cheesy but oh so true.

If your drinking has become problematic, it's likely there's not one area of your life that's not been affected negatively. If this isn't the case and you are simply interested in how to transition into a new era of your life that doesn't involve alcohol, then I am still willing to bet you will discover benefits you never would have thought of. Your work, relationships, finances and friendships will be better, all alongside your own physical and mental health. Remove booze, and there's not one area of your life that's not impacted in a positive way. I know this because I still live it and experience it and I also see this happening in the lives of so many others.

It's incredibly empowering seeing, feeling and living the improvements that you've created yourself because you decided to ditch just one thing. When you discover how to remove any hold or power alcohol has over you, you will come to see that in reality, all you are giving up is the monotony, the boredom, the predictability, the same old wine-stained shit, the hangovers, the irritability, the disappointment in yourself. And yet you are gaining so much potential in so many areas of your life. It's quite the trade-off!

You may well be shouting at me right now, 'But how the hell am I going to DO this?!' Don't worry – I am going to help you figure out the answer to that question (for you personally, as we are all different and I am not suggesting we all have the same relationship with booze or that what works for one person is necessarily right for another). I have been where you are. I totally understand your fears, worries and anxieties, but I also know you've 100 per cent got the power within you to change it all.

Perhaps the thought of never drinking alcohol again right now sounds overwhelming and out of reach. It might not even be something you particularly want to aim for at the moment and that's perfectly OK. It took me a good couple of years before I decided I was NEVER drinking again.

If you're reading this as a regular drinker who feels stuck in a rut, I've been where you are more times than I care to remember and the LAST thing I expected was to *not want* to drink again. For it to be a decision that I was happy, proud and confident to make, and to actually say it out loud when asked.

We all have a choice and my choice now is not to drink. In time, this might be yours too. Alcohol brings nothing positive to my life and I no longer want to drink. It's not a daily battle, it's not difficult, I just don't drink. It's that simple and yet it's liberating and brings untold freedom. Too much good stuff happened once I stopped and there's now no way on this planet that I would trade that for anything. Especially for something that would leave me worse off both mentally, physically AND in the pocket too!

"The greater the distance you put between yourself and that last drink you had, the more unwilling you become to compromise the positives"

But none of that has made me forget that it can feel hugely overwhelming to commit to a lifetime of sobriety. Which is why that's not something you need to do. What I am going to ask you to do though is to consider committing to 100 days booze-free. I'll explain more about the rationale behind this shortly, but since going sober, I've spoken to many people who've quit and almost everyone says that 100 days is the life-changing tipping point, when you will begin to look only forward, rather than back at your drinking days with rosé-tinted glasses. Don't worry if this seems like a lot right now. We're going to walk through it together.

Learning what life is like without booze – what *you* are like without regularly cracking a can or opening a bottle – is always going to be a valuable thing to do. It's just that 100 days is where the true life-changing magic begins to happen. The greater the distance you put between yourself and that last drink you had, the more unwilling you become to compromise the positives you're experiencing and the person you're beginning to unveil.

I once truly thought life without alcohol would be boring and not a single person could tell me any different. Had they even dared to try I wouldn't have listened to their utter nonsense anyway. Oh, the stuff I believed! The pedestal I placed alcohol on! The importance I gave it in my life! Sharing this with you now honestly makes me want to boil my own head because of how wrong I was! Life without alcohol is not boring – it's glorious, and if only I'd done it sooner. Alcohol well and truly had me in its grip, yet for so many wasted years I didn't even realise it.

Choice is everything. Not only is it OK to choose not to drink, it's a bloody wonderful and wholly liberating choice too. It's a choice that allows you to take back power and puts you in a place where phenomenal personal growth happens, because you're now able to finally discover who you are with complete clarity.

So if you're reading this as someone who's sober curious I implore you to give it a go. Don't lose another decade or two to living life below par, even as an occasional drinker who can take or leave it, when you could be experiencing the magic of an alcohol-free life. The first benefits will come quickly. The deeper, more unexpected changes will take longer and will likely require some hard work on your part, until the changes bed in and you don't want to drink any more, but it is so worth it. You absolutely have the power to turn everything around, you truly do.

BEN'S STORY

I didn't know that I needed to remove alcohol from my life completely when I decided to have a three-month break. I was the classic binge drinker. I wouldn't drink every day but once I'd started, I wouldn't stop. I'd get the first round in, drink mine in half the time it took everyone else to finish theirs, and the next round would be down on the table before anyone else had even thought about going to the bar.

I was a 'normal' drinker, I told myself, because everyone else I knew drank too. OK, maybe I was a *better* drinker than them, because I could put them away faster and handle more, but I certainly wasn't a 'problem' drinker.

Society tells us that problem drinkers are the people who drink every day – the 'vodka on the cereals' stereotype. They lose their jobs, their families and eventually themselves – whereas I had a good career, my family loved me (although their ever-growing concerns about my drinking had started to grate) and I was happy with who I was. But after starting one argument too many with my wife, Gem, after having one (or five) too many in the pub, I committed to a three-month break. And that was all it was ever meant to be.

But when I got to three months, I felt great. Gem, my parents, my brothers, my friends and my colleagues all told me I was doing great too. So, I decided to go for six months. And then twelve. Then on Day 366, I looked back at everything that I'd achieved over the last year without lager flowing through my veins and objectively decided that alcohol-free (AF) life was a good choice for me. Very simply, removing alcohol was helping me to fulfil my potential.

I don't know what would have happened if I'd carried on drinking. Would Gem have stuck with me? Would we have had our son, Leo? Would I have carried on slipping down the slippery slope, ignoring the deterioration of both my mental and physical health? I can't say for sure, but I can give it a firm 'probably'.

We can never know what the future holds. But without alcohol, I feel confident going into every day. Confident that I'll show up, do my best and deal with whatever happens with a clear head. I am proof that you don't need to have a rock bottom to decide to make a change and feel the benefits of life without alcohol.

If you've got that little voice in your head, like I did – listen to it. Because fulfilling your potential is more important than refilling your glass.

CHAPTER 2

'It's always gin o'clock somewhere!' (Me in 2018)

As we are going to be spending some time together, before we start the book proper, let me tell you a bit about me and the story of my relationship with alcohol.

I had my first taste of alcohol when I was in my early teens. I started to experiment with booze with school friends on a Friday and Saturday night: Cinzano drunk straight from the bottle, Special Brew poured down my throat while holding my nose and pretty much whatever we could get our hands on from our parents' drinks cabinets or get the older teenagers to buy us from the 'offy' (shorthand for off licence, or the liquor store). It definitely wasn't about the taste or a particular drink of choice; it was about drinking anything even barely palatable simply to get the desired effect, unpleasant as it was at first! It was vile stuff, which really should have been my first clue that this was not a good idea.

Loads of people my age were also trying alcohol for the first time and there was definitely a culture of teenagers with nothing much to do on a Friday night getting drunk in public places or at house parties. This served as my introduction to binge drinking – a habit that I sadly continued into my mid-forties.

I can't remember the first time I got drunk but I do remember one god-awful time when I was about fourteen or fifteen and my mum had come to collect me from a friend's house. We'd snaffled some of the cheapest and nastiest cider you could get your hands on and necked it while dossing about the streets. I was getting picked up from my friend's house around 10 o'clock at night and I just remember standing in her front room swaying in front of all these frowning adults, and being absolutely adamant we hadn't touched anything and we were all perfectly OK. It was the start of things to come, to be honest – thinking that drinking was a great idea until everything starts spinning but trying to bat it off with a convincing-enough 'I'M FINE', later confidently bragging 'I don't actually get hangovers, you know, I'm that good at drinking'. (Turns out, I was in a constant state of hangover for the best part of fifteen years.)

My teenage years weren't that different to those of a whole generation of experimenting kids. Maybe you were even one of them too, because it was so common growing up during the 1980s and 1990s. Drink, because everyone else is doing it.

I thought all my dreams had come true when best mate Jeanette and I rocked up at the Staffordshire University students' union and realised we could buy half a Carling for 50p! FIFTY FRIGGIN' PENCE! This was also the home of the hideous BLASTAWAY, available for a quid, which was a bottle of Castaway – a fruit-flavoured wine – mixed with a bottle of Diamond White cider. One pint of that and you were sorted for the night. Despite the availability of booze, though, my drinking wasn't problematic at uni and it certainly wasn't daily. I had an off switch in my twenties and a lot of the time I could take it or leave it – though somewhere between thirty and forty-four that switch got firmly stuck.

I'd finished uni with a decent degree in film, TV and radio then went on to successfully complete a postgraduate diploma in broadcast journalism. All I ever wanted to do was work in radio and at twenty-two I started working for a local commercial radio station. It was the absolute job of my dreams. And with it came party after party after party … I'd turn up to the opening of a new night club, a restaurant, an envelope. If there was free booze, I was there along with a load of like-minded party animals and we drank and drank and drank.

It's probably important to say at this point that I was always in charge of my own drinking. No one made me drink, no one really encouraged it, no one facilitated it and I didn't drink to block out trauma. I drank because I thought it was fun, because I thought it made *me* more fun. But those years of experimenting, which led to binge-drinking and drinking increased amounts more regularly, led me, slowly but surely, to becoming a daily drinking adult.

Sometimes problems can start precisely because something doesn't seem to be a problem. Because behaviour is normalised. When I was growing up, in northern England, no one batted an eyelid if you were necking a couple of tins in the sand dunes with a load of teenage mates – though thanks to the natural secrecy of teenagers, the adults didn't necessarily know we were doing it.

Equally, no one at uni thought it was weird to party your way through your three or four years there, guzzling cut-priced pints, because that's what everyone does, right? And of course you're going to socialise and network in your professional circle because it's expected, encouraged and for many years in my industry, it was paid for, so you'd be a mug if you didn't take advantage.

The changes in the way I drank happened very slowly and over a long period of time. During my thirties, I'd enjoy drinks with friends on nights out, I'd meet the girls for cocktails at a nice bar, I'd enjoy a glass of wine with dinner regularly and I'd look forward to weekends filled with family time, trips and probably Prosecco! At no point during these periods did I question my drinking or think there was even a glimmer of a problem. As I reached my late thirties and into my early forties, I saw no problem whatsoever with the regularity of my boozing.

And yet the truth was that I was becoming obsessed with booze. Yes, I was that knob on social media holding a large fishbowl of fruit-infused 'posh' gin up in the air declaring 'Chin, chin – it's 5 o'clock somewhere!', 'Happy Sunday!', 'Oh, I've earned THIS ONE!', ' … and RELAX!'. It makes my face ache just thinking about it now. Wherever possible, I would encourage others to join in and get wrecked with me. I would actively celebrate my ability to neck wine at speed at any given opportunity and I would drink whenever and wherever I could with whoever fancied it at the time. If they didn't, I'd do it solo.

Facebook Memories often remind me of just how mad my obsession with drinking got. Years ago, I went with friends on

"Changes happen very slowly and over a long period of time"

a Christmas shopping trip to The Trafford Centre on a Sunday afternoon, knowing full well I wasn't in the least bit interested in the shopping. I was fixated on just the drinking at the (s)wanky champagne bar. And there I was, within five minutes of the bar opening up at midday, raising some colourful and ridiculously overpriced cocktail in the air, taking a photo of the drink to share on my social media, making sure my newly manicured colourful nails were also in shot.

What an embarrassing crock of shit. For a start, no one cares. Not a single person. WHY do we do that? Why do we take photos of our drinks and share them with anyone we think is remotely interested? Bonkers, isn't it?

What the photo didn't show you was my bloated balloon face that was getting redder and more inflated as the years passed and the drinking increased. It didn't show you the anxiety starting to bubble knowing that tomorrow was already going to be a shit show – which I'd deal with by drinking more and worrying about that later. There is no 'after' shot taken seven hours later, showing me looking dead behind the eyes after a day-long drinking sesh. It didn't show me passing out on the settee at home later that night after topping up with more wine or vodka and it sure as hell didn't show you the misery I felt the day after the night before. It just showed you what I wanted people to see: booze = fun. Until it wasn't.

And as if the drinking wasn't all-consuming enough, I'd then have to plan the days after my drinking because I knew I'd feel like I'd been freshly dug up. I often feigned stomach upset or develop a mystery illness in the morning because I knew I couldn't drive on the school run. Truth was, I'd be utterly hanging and once again promising myself, while retching over the kids' breakfast, that ENOUGH WAS ENOUGH and there was no way I'd be drinking tonight. However, roll on 5 o'clock and I'd already be checking I had wine in the fridge and maybe some back-up spirits in the kitchen cupboard too. I mean, I couldn't possibly open a second bottle of Spanish rosé on a school night, so if there was gin or vodka behind the cereals I'd be reassured knowing I wouldn't run out.

Any social event was a signal to drink. A school fundraiser, a quiet 'quick one' on a sunny Sunday afternoon, the local village fete, a get-together with the girls, a mini-break away with the husband, a kid's birthday party, a shopping trip with friends. Every occasion started with a drink and ended with me either peaking too soon, making a prize Drunken Dick of myself, passing out, disappearing for a tactical chunder so I could make room for more booze, having to go home early or simply falling asleep. I was becoming more and more reliant on a painfully addictive substance that was very much not loving me back.

Looking back and knowing what I know now, I could have saved myself a whole decade of increased drinking, blackouts and crippling hangovers if I'd found the courage to speak to someone, to put my hand up or to admit my drinking levels were slowly but surely increasing. But because alcohol is SO celebrated and so normalised I didn't pay it enough attention and simply kept going. Ignorance is bliss, right?!

But on some level, I knew this couldn't go on. Did I want to carry on like this, watching the clock and counting down until I could crack open the wine and then really ramp it up at weekends? Did I *really* have a problem? (While I was in the thick of it and waist deep in rosé, I genuinely did not realise how bad it had got.) I was oblivious at this point in my life that I had the power to change absolutely everything with one simple yet huge decision. To not drink.

I eventually decided, in my forties, that it was probably a good idea to take an occasional break. So I'd attempt the occasional Sober October or Dry January. In June 2018, I decided I'd do twenty-eight days of no booze – though I'd already decided I was drinking again on 1 July – and for the most part, I 'enjoyed' it. Which may sound surprising, but, realistically, you can't NOT enjoy waking up feeling fresh, getting stuff done and feeling proud that for once you're not giving in to alcohol at every given opportunity. I was aware that everything felt … better. Don't get me wrong, it was HARD, but it also set me up nicely for what was to come just a couple of months later.

As hard as it was and despite the fact I began to learn more about what life could potentially be like without alcohol being the constant focal point, I was NOT considering forever at this point, it wasn't even on my radar, but I was thinking about a longer period of time off the booze. Deep down, I knew I quite liked not drinking, but I hadn't really fathomed WHY. Because it was such a big part of who I was – or so I'd told myself – once July rolled around, I was going to get back on it, keep drinking

"I had the power to change absolutely everything with one simple yet huge decision: to not drink" through the summer and THEN set a date for a ninety-day break. No ifs. No buts. No excuses. No alcohol for ninety days. A three-month break from the booze to reset, to get my very drunk ducks in a row, to learn how to moderate (lolz!), and to show my family and friends that I could return to a new way of drinking by controlling it after a sensible – but probably miserable as shit – extended dry stint.

So that's what I did: I set yet *another* date for a break after yet *another* summer of drinking. Even though I was nervous at the prospect, a teeny-weeny little part of me hidden somewhere deep down in the wobbly wine belly was sort of looking forward to it. I'd felt really good in June, then I proceeded to undo all my hard work in July and August. Truthfully, I was knackered and sick and tired of feeling sick and tired. So I bit the bullet and set a date for ninety days of no booze, utterly oblivious to the fact that Monday, 3 September 2018 would be the start of the most magical, life-changing journey.

I didn't know it in part because the Monday morning hangover was bordering on death – the retching painful, the anxiety crippling and the thought of ever drinking alcohol again utterly spew-inducing. Even thinking back to that hangover after a Sunday of day drinking in the sunshine – that ended with me crying for no reason in a friend's back garden and then passing out on their settee – gives me the shivers. The joy of knowing I never have to feel like that again is priceless.

OVER THE INFLUENCE

One of the things I'm most proud of in my life – aside from my three children, obviously! – is the online community I set up to connect people who had or wanted to quit drinking. In 2020, I started a podcast called 'Over the Influence' with my friend Ben Anderson, all about living and navigating life alcohol-free. The community and support group grew from this – all helping each other on our varied journeys, talking openly about our relationship with alcohol in a non-judgemental space.

It happened organically and it certainly wasn't part of some Big Sober Plan. It came about because people asked for it, because people wanted to connect, share and celebrate their sobriety with each other. It grew because it turns out that although you can feel like you have to tackle sobriety alone, or that there is something embarrassing about giving up drinking, like there is something wrong with you, the opposite is true. There are many people all in the same boat, willing to talk, to share, to help. And to embrace all the joyful things that come about when you quit alcohol. We now have members across the globe from the UK to Europe, from New Zealand to Venezuela and from Canada to the States. It's incredible and sometimes I have to pinch myself to confirm that all this is happening because I decided it was time to take an extended break from booze.

On the podcast, we chat to people who've had real rock bottoms and who've *had* to stop drinking to ultimately save themselves; to authors whose books have changed our lives and those of many of our listeners; we meet the Instagrammers and the TikTokkers who are inspiring and influencing thousands and we also talk to ordinary people now doing extraordinary things simply because they decided to change just one thing in their lives, often with the most beautiful of results. Some of my favourite episodes are with our own community members who've hit a year and beyond alcohol-free, and who want to let people like you know it's so worth sticking with as they too have finally discovered the life-changing magic of quitting alcohol.

I'll talk a bit more about this community in particular, as well as the importance of communities in general when you make a big life change, in a few pages time. This for me is the best example of how remarkable things can come about when you choose to say no to booze, though I have plenty of other examples too. I can't wait for you to give it a try and find out what it might make space for in your life.

CHAPTER 3

. . . .

Tell me about this 'magic' …

n the UK and other countries where drinking is a routine, accepted part of the culture, where special events are toasted with champagne or a celebratory round down the pub, and 'raising a glass' is just what you do, then it's natural to wonder how you are going to socialise, date, go on holiday, celebrate or even connect with people without booze. Well, surprisingly, it's actually often easier than you think, and we are going to get on to how you do it. But first of all, let's start by looking at some of the magic that you can expect in a life without alcohol.

YOUR PHYSICAL HEALTH IMPROVES

'Yes, yes, alcohol is bad for you. Tell me something I don't know, Sharon,' I hear you say. But until you try it, you probably don't know how much better you can feel in your own body when you're not asking it to process a substance that is, frankly, poisonous, on a regular or semi-regular basis.

You may find your bloated beach-ball balloon face deflates, your egg-on-legs belly changes shape, the bright whites return to your eyes and your skin takes on the kind of radiance that makes people ask if you have been on holiday. All these things are on the cards, but what is certain is that you will have more energy and you are far more likely to make good decisions that will impact your wider health.

Maybe you're a budding marathon runner who really wants to ditch the booze and focus on your training, or maybe you are about as inclined to go out for a jog as you are to fly to the moon. It doesn't matter. You are far less likely to bail on that family walk, eat your body weight in carbs or stay up way later than you intended when you are not boozing or feeling groggy from the night before.

YOU'RE DOING YOUR MENTAL HEALTH A HUGE FAVOUR

If drinking is prompting you to question your own relationship with alcohol, if it's making you feel anxious in the days afterwards, if it's being mentioned by friends and family who care about you or if it's simply making you feel like shit, then you're doing the right thing by picking up this book and starting to work towards an alcohol-free life.

But even if you don't relate to these scenarios particularly, your brain is still highly likely to feel the benefits of ditching booze. Colour returns to your world, the laughter gets louder, the sky is bluer, the once-annoying dawn chorus rings clearer. Imagine never waking up with that creeping fear of *Was I awful last night?*

"There's no more waking up with a blinding headache or even a dull throb"

You'll also never have to question whether how you feel is being influenced by what you drank. If you feel anxious then that's something you can work on, rather than going round in circles wondering if it's mainly the bottle of wine you sunk the previous night giving you the panics. If you feel like skipping along the road and breaking into song, that's because you are happy and it's not the giddy warmth of a few glasses of fizz sloshing around your system.

YOU'LL NEVER HAVE ANOTHER HANGOVER

I'm stating the blindingly obvious here but one of the first benefits you're going to feel straight away is having a clear head in the morning. You're not going to wake up with a blinding headache or even a dull throb. You're also not going to be unnaturally thirsty because you'll be hydrated. Imagine that – starting every day feeling normal, fresh and well, with a head that doesn't need tending to with painkillers alongside breakfast!

Having proudly woken up with a clear head since my own sobriety, I know, hand on heart, that I'll never experience the horrors of a crippling hangover ever again – the headache, the nausea, the sweating, the aches, the thirst, the insomnia, the memory loss, the subsequent junk food and then the inevitable large wine later on to take the edge off leading to the whole sorry misery-go-round once more. No. Thank. You. It's such a freeing feeling knowing I won't ever have to battle through another hangover, especially as they lasted longer the older I got.

YOUR RELATIONSHIPS IMPROVE

Maybe you know quite a few people who don't, or rarely, drink, or maybe the main thing that has been holding you back from trying out an alcohol-free life is the reactions from friends and not knowing how you are going to navigate a sober social life. If it's the latter, then don't worry – we are going to come on to this. What I want to say here is that your friendships change and become more meaningful and you are likely to be more fun for your family to be around too. For example, I found was much less shouty at the kids because I felt better in the mornings, plus I DID more with them because I wasn't counting down to wine o'clock.

Yes, there might be a few people who don't get it at first, and there may be a few hurdles to overcome, but this is a chance to make sure you have real relationships based on fun, friendship and trust, rather than a mutual appreciation of happy hour and booze-fuelled oversharing.

YOUR BANK BALANCE WILL THANK YOU

It's not just the amount you hand over in return for a glass or bottle of something, is it? It's the taxi home, the takeaway you didn't really need, the carby snacks you buy the next day to keep you going when you are tired from a late night and/or a hangover from too much booze. You might not want to consider the sum right now but trust me, when you realise that this money can

"Friendships change and become more meaningful"

be allocated to other things – to treats that make you happy but always seem too indulgent or towards your long-term financial goals – it's a great motivator.

I still use an app called I Am Sober to track what I would have been spending and I reckon I was spending around an extra £8.50 a day. This conservative figure doesn't account for increased spending on drinks at weekends in bars, pubs or restaurants, taxis, junk food or buying rounds. So far, in the time since I have given up drinking – DRUM ROLL, PLEASE – I'm looking at a saving of around £20,000. I'll say it again … that's TWENTY THOUSAND POUNDS I have chosen not to spend on alcohol. Mind blowing, isn't it?

YOU GET TO KNOW YOURSELF BETTER

How many times have you heard it said that being drunk reveals exactly who are? It's the biggest crock of shite I've ever heard. Alcohol makes you say and do things you wouldn't even consider when sober. You want to know the surefire way to find out exactly who you are? Stop drinking, strap in, hold on and enjoy the ride! It won't be too long before you're reaping those little rewards and enjoying those well-deserved pangs of pride when you realise this life you're carving out for yourself is made possible because you're repeatedly making the decision to say no to alcohol and yes to being yourself – even when it's hard.

If your experience is even a bit like mine, I bet that you will find that your confidence increases, you grasp new challenges with clarity and excitement, you say yes to what you love and no to the people-pleasing shite of the past. You start to grow, your world gets bigger, the foggy lid of dull, grey clouds is lifted and the sparkle that you once had begins to peep through and eventually shines brighter than ever before. You start to live authentically and proudly in ways you probably can't even imagine right now.

If you are a regular drinker, and particularly if you use alcohol as a way to deal with social situations, stripping away the layers of alcohol which have been building up over the years like a huge sticking plaster reveals the true you underneath. Even though it can be hard and uncomfortable at times it's also quite the revelation and the only way to really know yourself properly, in my view.

· · ·

When you stop drinking, your life improves immeasurably. That's not to say the daily grind doesn't continue – of course it does – but it's how you *deal* with life and all it throws at you that changes. My life has got bigger in ways I could only have dreamt of more than six years ago. In ways I didn't even know I wanted it to. In ways I literally could have never imagined. Stopping drinking isn't about what you're 'giving up', it's about everything you gain. So while it's natural to feel trepidation or even doubt, I want you to try to allow yourself to get excited about all these benefits that are waiting for you down the road when you take control and stop letting booze take up space it doesn't deserve.

"When you stop drinking, your life improves immeasurably"

ANDY'S STORY

Ten years ago I proudly defined myself as a drinker. It served me in my late teens and twenties, but in my thirties, my drinking changed when I became a husband and father with responsibilities. I became reliant on it to take the edge off a difficult day and I thought it made parenting easier.

As I turned forty I knew I had to make a change. I ran two marathons while drinking heavily trying to prove to myself and my family that all was OK. Sadly, it was not. Running the London Marathon in 2017 was followed by a deep low period where my alcohol consumption and poor choices when drunk escalated. I checked out on my responsibilities as a father, a husband and a business owner. I did not like the person I'd become. It was time for change.

I found an online community and quietly went about the process of trying to change my relationship with alcohol. It took me almost a year of trying to break the cycle. I thought it was impossible but eventually, in March 2019, something clicked and I had my last drink. This was over five years ago.

I carried a lot of shame in the early days of being alcohol-free (AF). Why could I not be normal? Why could I not be trusted to have a drink? Why was I the one with the problem?

I now know who I am. I have learned to be in full control of my actions, I've discovered a clarity I never knew existed, I've developed deeper connections, I've become so much more consistent with my actions and I'm content. All because I gave up one thing and gained so much more. The biggest things it has brought me are self-compassion and learning to like myself again. What a gift.

Life now is so different. I am proud to be AF and want to share the joys with anyone that's prepared to listen. I've run ten marathons and three five-day ultra events. My fitness is the best it's ever been in my life. I'm 30kg lighter and running faster than ever as I approach my fiftieth birthday. I have my own AF runners community and I am proud to be helping others find the joys of AF living through coaching. My children have grown up not knowing their dad as a drinker. They can see that they know there is a choice – something I never knew.

Removing alcohol doesn't automatically make life perfect because it still throws you curveballs (I was diagnosed with prostate cancer in 2023), but it means that you are so much more likely to have the tools to deal with whatever happens. Life is just so much easier.

I feel so lucky to have been a problematic drinker who had to go through pain to discover a new way of living – one where giving up one thing would result in gaining so much. The future feels exciting. There is so much I want to achieve in this one precious life.

CHAPTER 4

· · · · · · · · · · · · · ·

How do I know if I have a problem?

ESSENTIAL HEALTH WARNING

*If you are physically addicted to alcohol, or think you might be, then it is **absolutely essential** to see your doctor or a qualified medical professional. Stopping drinking suddenly when there is a physical dependency can be very dangerous, and may even be fatal if you are not supervised professionally through a medical withdrawal.*

Please don't let shame or stigma stop you from asking for help. I really hope that the joy of being booze-free that I describe in these pages helps to inspire you, but as I think you probably know already, you are going to need a few people in your corner – not just me in book form – so please, please get the help you need. You absolutely CAN do this.

One of the many, many things alcohol demands of you is mental energy. When was the last time you:

- Compared your drinking habits to someone else's, because you felt anxious about your own or to reassure yourself that you don't drink *that* much or *that* often?

- Did a deal with yourself about how much you were 'allowed' to drink on a certain night?

- Broke the deal you made with yourself or drank more than you had thought you would?

- Spent more money on a night out than you wanted to?

- Changed your plans as a result of drinking – for example, cancelled plans with friends or family, or skipped the exercise you were intending to do?

- Took an online test or just googled the words 'Am I an alcoholic?' out of curiosity?

If you are having these thoughts even semi-regularly then at the very least that gets kind of exhausting, right?

I've just typed 'Am I an' into Google and 'Am I an alcoholic' is the first suggestion that appears. So if you have asked this question of a search engine then you're definitely not the first person to do it and you certainly won't be the last! At the time of writing, there are 2,620,000,000 results listed for that single search alone. This is the first thing I read:

'Common signs of alcoholism include: Wanting to stop drinking but can't. Drinking more than intended, or binge drinking. Spending a significant amount of time and money on alcohol use. Continuing alcohol use even though it's causing problems with your life and health.'

Scroll a bit further and you can get all your answers by clicking on 'Our Alcoholic Quiz Can Help You Find Out!', followed by the '10 Warning Signs of Alcoholism' and rounded off with another fun-sounding quiz – the 'Alcoholism Self Test'! Joy! What better way to spend half an hour on the sofa while crying into your pinot.

Let me tell you something: you're much better off asking *yourself* if you've got a drinking problem, rather than the internet. The most important question isn't whether you fill some external criteria of 'person with a drinking problem' but if alcohol is causing problems in *your* life. Is it stopping you from living to your fullest, happiest potential?

That's not to say there's not a ton of useful information available out there that might help you, of course there is, but there's also a load of information (and, let's face it, misinformation!) that might make you feel worse and, in turn, push you to drink more or simply hide from what you're trying to work out in the first place.

So rather than ask the internet if you're an alcoholic, just step back, ask yourself a couple of questions and answer honestly:

- How happy are you with alcohol in your life?
- Is drinking causing you problems? If so, in what way?
- What in your life is likely to improve without alcohol in it?

I know many people who will openly admit they were addicted to booze and plenty more who absolutely were not but could identify that their drinking habits had changed in a way that they weren't comfortable with. The spectrum of drinking is vast – from someone who can have a couple one weekend and then not bother for a month to someone who has become physically addicted and needs a safe, supervised medical withdrawal.

It doesn't matter where you place yourself on that spectrum. If you want to change your relationship with alcohol, you can. Plus, it's worth remembering that it's SO much easier to address any concerns you may have while you're still in control and before alcohol has the chance to get its claws in a bit deeper.

One of the first steps to take in order to experience the life-changing magic of quitting alcohol is to acknowledge how bad it's got for YOU ... if indeed it has. You might not feel it's *that* bad – but there's no reason on earth why you have to wait for it to get worse! Drinking doesn't have to be affecting your day-to-day life negatively; your life with alcohol doesn't need to be a drunken disaster zone. Always remember that you don't need a rock bottom in order to reassess your drinking and decide to change your relationship with alcohol. You can just simply choose to stop!

I have found that friends, family, neighbours, colleagues, acquaintances and even strangers have been fascinated when they have found out that I choose not to drink alcohol. Among the questions I get, one that used to crop up often was along the lines of 'How bad did it get?' In other words, what terrible calamity did I inflict on myself before I was forced to call it a day. This question – however it is phrased – has been put to me by a whole host of people who assume they've got the right to know. Let's set this straight from the start: they don't! It's a very personal thing to ask and, to be honest, it's my business and no one else's.

The question was often posed by drinkers who wanted to measure their own alcohol consumption against mine to check

"You can just simply choose to stop!"

how 'problematic' their drinking may or may n̄.. people were simply curious; some were utterly baffl̄. were those who were genuinely concerned about ....al health and wellbeing. There were also drinkers who wanted to share with me honestly and confidentially that they too had found themselves drinking more, and more regularly, or even seeking out wine or spirits that were slightly higher in ABV (alcohol by volume) to get drunk more quickly and effectively.

But this question – be it curious, probing or blunt – is a reminder of how ingrained alcohol is in society, how it's at the centre of just about everything we do for enjoyment, celebration or commiseration and how it's the only drug in the world you find yourself justifying NOT taking when you decide to cut down, take a break or remove it from your life altogether. This is what underpins the idea that you have to be forced to give up, that you would only stop drinking if you had no choice. Whereas the opposite is true!

Imagine saying to someone you had given up coffee because it was giving you a headache – or even just because you thought it was too expensive. Almost anyone would agree that was a good idea. You wouldn't wait until your daily espresso was causing you migraines and insomnia before you packed it in, would you?

I love this quote from the Scottish actor and comedian Billy Connolly: 'I decided to quit drinking while it was still my idea.' You and me both, Billy! Although I wasn't fully physically addicted to alcohol I was certainly physically and mentally dependent on it, and it was a habit that I was struggling to change the more the years went on. It never ceases to amaze me how many people want to tell me THEY HAVEN'T GOT A PROBLEM because they only drink at weekends and never in the week, or that they don't touch spirits and only stick to wine or beer. Booze is booze regardless of the packaging, ABV percentage or day of the week, and you can still have a problematic or dependent relationship with alcohol even if your drinking is confined to 'only' at the weekends or monthly binges.

I asked some of our Over the Influence community members if they'd ever taken any of these online quizzes or asked the internet 'Have I got a drinking problem?', and how that worked out for them. This is what a few of them shared:

SUZANNE – 'I googled something along the lines of "Am I an alcoholic?" and did answer quizzes but they weren't helpful, really. I think you read into it what you want to, anyway – in my case, "See, you're fine!" When actually it doesn't matter how much you drink compared to others, it matters how you feel about it.'

JONNY – 'Yes! Because I wondered if I was an alcoholic. Even though no one bar me would see the result, I felt shit about it. So I went for a pint or six. Asking Google the question didn't help on its own. It was just another building block in me making a case for myself that eventually led me to quit.'

HELEN – 'I did google that dreaded question when I knew I needed to stop. It confirmed what I knew anyway, which is

"Alcoholism is a disease, not a character flaw"

that I was drinking way too much, it was putting me at risk of alcohol-related health issues and impacting my life. But the label of 'alcoholic' was not necessary or helpful and I was holding it together/"functioning". I felt worried, I think. And I felt shame. I hid it like I hid a proportion of my drinking.'

Ultimately, what's important is how alcohol is making you *feel* and not just the amount or regularity of your drinking.

Years ago, I connected with a woman online and we would discuss our drinking habits. She's the loveliest person and shared with me that she was trying to stop her one-glass-a-night red wine habit. And that's all it was: a single glass of wine each night with dinner. She wasn't physically addicted to alcohol. There was no rock bottom. She wasn't upsetting her friends and family. At first, I thought she was bonkers. I used to DREAM of having 'just one'. Just one glass instead of at least one bottle. Her drinking was where I'd have loved mine to be: moderate and controlled without turning her into a vomiting, noisy mess. Yet, that one glass of red wine a night, my lovely friend had decided, was too much *for her*. She didn't like how it made her feel, how it had become habitual, and she wanted to stop drinking it, simple as that. And you know what? She asked herself the tough question of whether alcohol was causing her problems, and she decided that removing that relatively small amount of alcohol from her life would change her life immeasurably, which it did. She was less snappy with family, had more energy in the morning and felt better all round.

To her, drinking that amount daily was a problem. So she did something about it.

If booze is causing you problems – however big or small – it's OK to admit that. In fact, it's important to do so, as it's hard to solve a problem you can't name. It's not about putting a label on yourself. It's not admitting defeat and telling the world you're an alcoholic. As an aside, though, it's really important to acknowledge that for a huge number of people, using the word alcoholic *is* incredibly helpful and it helps them remain sober. Alcoholism is a disease, not a character flaw.

It's also worth acknowledging here that there's a difficulty in asking yourself if you've got a drinking problem, as in many ways, it's not always possible to fully grasp or admit where alcohol might have taken you until you stop for an extended period of time. For example, if hangovers, general tiredness and/or low mood after a big weekend are normal for you, you may even have stopped noticing and not even realise how much better you could feel. I *suspected* I might have an issue but genuinely didn't realise quite how bad it had got until I stopped and I was able to look back in the rear view mirror. Hindsight is a wonderful thing and my only regret is not giving myself a chance sooner.

So I am going to say it one more time here: you DO NOT NEED TO WAIT until you suspect you may have a drinking problem in order to change your relationship with alcohol. You can do it now and save yourself a stack of money, time and worry. If alcohol has any role in your life at all – main character, supporting artist, occasional cameo – you can STILL stop drinking and enjoy the magic of an alcohol-free life. It's SO much better to be asking questions of your drinking early. Don't do what I did and ignore the voice for a decade!

You might be feeling nervous in acknowledging that alcohol is causing you problems at whatever level but I hope you might also be feeling a tiny bit excited at the prospect of having the power to change the path of your life in ways you could only dream of – if you give yourself the chance you deserve and make some lifestyle changes.

"You do not need to wait

CHAPTER 5

. . . .

Can I learn to moderate my drinking?

don't know – can you? How has that been working out for you so far?

If I could moderate, I would've done so years ago and saved myself a whole load of time, money and hangovers! The number of people who've said to me, 'Oh Shaz, just have one!' even while knowing full well what I was like as a drinker and having seen firsthand that 'just one' for me would mean one bottle. I've never managed 'just one' of anything, to be honest, but these days it's coffee, Creme Eggs and Magnums (the ice creams on sticks, not magnums of booze!).

That's not to say people *can't* moderate – the world is full of natural moderators. You may well consider yourself one of them and if that's the case I applaud you – but when it comes to alcohol, I've spoken to enough guests on the Over the Influence podcast, sober friends and community members to know that moderation also doesn't exist for them and is virtually impossible for anyone who's had any sort of issue with alcohol previously. This is because:

a) It's an addictive substance

b) It's progressive, as in the more you drink, the more your body eventually needs to get that one-or-two glass buzz.

The purpose of this book isn't to debate moderation or work out a complicated way where we can somehow keep *a bit* of booze in our lives ... it's to celebrate sobriety in all its raw and unexpected glory and to give you an insight into how truly magical life can be as a non-drinker. So I would suggest that moderators too could massively benefit from removing alcohol and experiencing the magic of sobriety! You do not need to be a problematic drinker, an alcoholic or binge drinker to qualify – it applies to absolutely everyone. Just because you can have one glass and leave it, doesn't mean you have to or even want to!

When you've previously thought about cutting down, having a dry spell or removing alcohol completely, have you ever said to yourself, 'I shall moderate my drinking, drink only on "special" occasions and that will be the end of that'? How did it make you feel? Did you find yourself setting rules to make your drinking more controlled? I'll give you a sneaky peak into how moderation looked for ME – though I'd really like to stress again that some people are able to moderate.

When I tried to moderate it really revealed that I did have problem with alcohol. The NOISE that moderation caused in my head was deafening and rather than helping with my drinking, it made it a whole lot worse, not least because of the ridiculous List of Moderation Rules I'd find myself making each time I wanted to drink for a special occasion (it's amazing how fast those 'special occasions' came round!) or event that I couldn't *possibly* enjoy without a glass of something in my hand. It went something like this: 'OK, so the event is on Saturday, I definitely, 100 per cent won't drink this week. Actually, I won't touch a drop until Saturday and I'll also have Friday off and "save myself" for the weekend. I'll just stick to wine, three large glasses max AND I'll be super good and have soft drinks in between. That way I won't get drunk too quickly, I'll remain relatively hydrated AND I'll be able to function Sunday too. Easy.'

This is the plan I usually had in my head the week before. I never, ever followed it. Setting up the rules always led to failure, usually by the Tuesday of that week. In many ways, it caused me to fixate on drinking even more. I'd then start to renegotiate my own rules with myself, reasoning that actually, come Friday, I could just have a couple ahead of the event, and ONLY a couple. It's the start of the weekend after all! Again, I'll eat well, not drink on an empty stomach and stick to one type of alcohol.

And then there were the rules I'd attempt to make for drinking at home. I'll only have one. Probably a large one, but just one nonetheless. I'll not have spirits, only at weekends. I won't drink on my own, only in the company of others. If the booze runs out, I won't buy any more. And so it went on and on and on …

The noise was relentless and the more I tried to moderate the louder the noise got and the more I set myself up to fail.

I remember hearing the story of a member from our Over the Influence community who left the group for a short while because he wanted to return to moderate drinking. After an extended break from booze, he was feeling confident that he had it under control and he was going to pick and choose the occasions when he would drink. He was sure that these occasions were only going to be the 'special' ones. But soon enough, the speed at which those 'special occasions' came around was quicker than he realised. He began looking for excuses to turn any event into something 'special' so he could validate his drinking. And before he knew it, those problematic drinking levels returned. That was the penny drop moment for him, and he knew then he didn't want to drink anymore.

If any of this resonates with you, have a think about the rules you might have made for yourself about your drinking. When you're going to drink. What you're going to drink. Where you're going to drink. Who you're going to drink with. How you're going to drink. The amount you're going to drink.

What I'm getting at here is that doesn't the fact you've even MADE rules throw up a red flag in itself? If you've not got a drinking problem, would you need the rules?

Noisy, isn't it?

Shutting the door firmly on alcohol for a set period of time – and I mean slammed shut with not a chink of light showing through and the door temporarily locked – removes that noise, introduces silence where the booze would have been and gives you space to think about all the other things you'd like to do instead of drink. Don't get me wrong, that silence at first can be deafening! But it doesn't last, you get stronger with each passing day and alcohol becomes far less important with time.

"You get stronger with each passing day and alcohol becomes far less important with time"

I tried, and for many years I'd give Sober October a good go – some years I even did the whole month (yay me!). I just hadn't cemented WHY I wanted to do this – as you started to do in the previous chapter – and was still too obsessed with boozing to take the time to work it out and give a shit.

If this is you now, taking the odd extended break here and there, then bloody good on you. It's where it starts and it all counts.

If you can confidently say that you're a 'just one' type of drinker, you can take or leave it, for the time being, you're going to leave it. If your drinking looks more like mine in terms of volume and frequency, if you feel comfortable in doing so, you should feel no embarrassment in admitting you struggle to have just one so you're trying life with none.

In my experience, none is SO much easier than one anyway as it removes that whole moderation quandary. 'Just one' allows the door to remain ajar a little bit which means the strong possibility of another drink and then another after that. 'None' closes it firmly shut, even if you're a moderate drinker simply curious about what alcohol-free life might look like for you. No internal negotiations are needed with none. It's simpler, it's effective and it stops the noise for as long as you decide.

And it is for you to decide. Which you don't need to do now. No one is asking you to get up and declare to all and sundry 'I am NEVER drinking again!'. All you need to do is make a plan, make a start and keep choosing to say no to a drink for as long as you decide to.

So let's begin.

KELLY'S STORY

Drinking alcohol became an issue for me in 2015.
I wasn't coping with life's stresses and I was suffering
with bulimia. Alcohol went from being fun at the
weekends to my almost daily coping mechanism.
My self-esteem was so low and I wasn't being my true
self as I didn't think I was good enough. This led me
to telling a lot of lies and ultimately not living in line
with my values, which in turn made me hate myself
even more.

In July 2021, I joined the Over the Influence (OTI)
community after listening to the podcast. My drinking
had ramped up during lockdown and I was fed up of
feeling tired, sluggish and full of anxiety. I knew that
alcohol was holding me back in so many areas of my
life and it was badly affecting my mental health. I was
really nervous at the start. I would join Zooms calls but
would keep my camera off. But I started to become
more comfortable and I realised I had nothing to be
nervous about.

I was managing a few weeks sober at a time but kept
falling back into the same boring cycle. However,
now, each time I gave in to temptation my alcohol
consumption increased, my mental health worsened
and, in turn, I hated myself even more.

In September 2021, I decided this was it. I had to make changes and put the work in to stay sober and started interacting with fellow OTI members on Zooms.

I would love to say that I have been alcohol-free since then but unfortunately between then and February 2022 my life slowly began to fall apart. However, through the support on Zooms and in the forum along with the friendships I have made as part of a sober community, I'm now approaching two years sober and I'm the strongest I've ever been.

I now run marathons for fun, I consistently show up in work and, most importantly, my three sons have their mum back. A mum who is patient, reliable and always there for them, day or night.

I have started training to become an alcohol-free coach so that I can hopefully help people who are starting out on their alcohol-free journey and might be struggling like I did. I am actively taking steps to progress my career into a role that has been a long-time aspiration and hopefully in all of this I am being a good role model to my boys, showing them that you can achieve anything in life that you put your mind to.

CHAPTER 6

What do I want to be different?

So, as we've established, it's pretty soul-destroying to be sitting by yourself on the settee late at night drinking while asking the phone in your hand if you've got a drinking problem. And it's not going to achieve anything. So instead, we need to take a look at the ways in which drinking is a negative thing for you personally and then focus on what would be different if you removed it.

As I think we all are aware, alcohol so often brings with it a lot of negative emotions. Shame. Feeling like shit. Depression. Confusion. Embarrassment. This list goes on. I mean, that's probably one of the reasons you're here, right? Who wants that in their life?

At this point, I am going to ask you to think about the problems alcohol causes you personally and ask you to write them down. I'm sorry if this feels difficult or confronting. It is important to understand what it is that we want to remove from our lives so we can crack on and make a plan to do just that. Try to be as honest as you can. You don't have to write it here on the page – get a separate piece of paper if that feels better.

Just remember, that this is a difficult first step on an important journey that is going to take you to a magical place. Once it's done, you will be closer to experiencing the magic of a life without booze. Here are some prompts to help you think about the problems alcohol might be causing you.

- What worries you most about your relationship with alcohol?

- What problems are caused when you drink?
  (Are they big problems concerning relationships, friendships, work, home or finances, or smaller issues that bubble away in the background? Many people would say it's a mixture of both ...)

- What do you think you are missing out on because of alcohol?

- How would you feel if you were able to make moves towards solving these problems completely?

As I mentioned before, if you've been habitually drinking for years, as I had, that's your normal and you probably will struggle to envisage all the positives that would come from not drinking. So discover on the following pages some areas that will almost certainly improve when you remove alcohol. Take a moment to think about each one and what they would look like for you.

"Alcohol is a thief of energy and time"

Here are some opening questions for you to consider, if you removed alcohol from your life:

- How would you feel?
- What could you do that you can't or don't do now?
- What wider implications would this have for you?
- What wider implications would this have for the people around you?

ENERGY

Even drinking relatively small amounts of booze as you get older can leave you feeling flat and lacking in energy the day after the night before, or a bit washed out and cranky because you stayed up late and had another, even though you'd promised yourself earlier you weren't going to. Alcohol is a thief of energy and time and when it's removed, no matter what your levels of drinking might look like, you get both back in abundance.

What could you do with more time and energy?

MOTIVATION

When you have more energy, you're likely to have more motivation. You begin to tackle the small jobs you might have put off because you've got more time and inclination to do so. You become more productive as not only are you filling the gaps where you may have previously been drinking, you are never hungover or left feeling dull or low because of what you drank the day before. Do not underestimate the effect that booze can have on your inclination to get shit done, even a few days after you've had a couple of glasses on a school night.

What might you do with a bit more get up and go?

FINANCES

This might be a fun one. What would you like to spend the cash on if you didn't spend it in the pub or bar, or on stocking up the booze cupboard? Even if you are not a big drinker, this can still add up over time.

How much do you currently spend on booze?

RELATIONSHIPS

How much of your focus do you give to alcohol? Do you avoid being Parent Taxi and resent the family doing stuff later on in the day because it's eating into your Wine Time? Are you letting friends and family down and prioritising drinking over other activities? Are you looking at the clock and counting down to when you feel it's acceptable to have a drink? Have you cancelled or postponed plans because you've felt tired and a bit below par? Or 'phoned it in' with friends or loved ones because you felt a bit shady after a few pints the night before?

Which relationships in your life would you like to dedicate a bit more time and energy to, and how might ditching the booze help that?

HEALTH

It's amazing how simply choosing not to drink can have a wide-ranging impact on your health. Even if you basically replace the calories with cake, as I do, it's still highly likely that you will feel better. It's not just that you aren't asking your body to devote resources to clearing the toxins you put in it. You're much less likely to eat food that's bad for you when you're not pissed or hungover. That extra motivation might get you to the gym or out for a hike. When you look in the mirror and realise you've lost the bloat, the eye bags are now small rucksacks rather than suitcases and you look like you've had a facial without having to have a facial, you'll feel better as a result, which will likely create a positive feedback loop where it's easy to make good choices for your health because *this* is now your normal and you always want to feel like this.

Would you like to feel brighter and healthier and pain-free?

THE HEALTH BENEFITS OF NO BOOZE

What are the things that spring to mind when you imagine your health and wellbeing when it's not under the shadow of booze?

For me, I didn't realise how calm I would feel. How my loud, shouty voice became quieter when trying to get the kids to listen. I felt a patience I didn't know I was capable of in all aspects of my life. The mysterious aches, pains and throbs disappeared along with my frustation and my overall health and wellbeing just levelled up naturally.

If you're functioning at around a 7 out of 10 right now, imagine yourself being a solid 9 or 10. What's changed? How are you feeling? How are you making others close to you feel? This is a really good time to ask yourself WHY you want to do this. If you're struggling a bit thinking about your reasons, don't worry, because we're going to work through this together in the next chapter. It's a Big Question!

"When you have more energy, you're likely to have more motivation"

CHAPTER 7

· · · · · · · · · · · · ·

What's my 'why'?

Part of the reason that the few forays I made into giving up drinking for Sober October or Dry January weren't particularly successful was that I hadn't really sat down and thought about WHY I wanted to give up. I found it hard to face the truth of where drinking was getting me and I didn't focus on what not drinking might bring me.

So, before we get started on making a plan, I'd like to encourage you to ask yourself a really simple question – WHY? Why do you want to stop drinking? What are your reasons for wanting to make a change?

It may be the case that you have one reason only. Or you may have several reasons including your mental health, your physical health, your family, your career. What matters is what's important to *you*.

At this point in time, you might not feel ready to stop drinking, but taking some time to think it through and nailing down your 'why's might just help you work out where you are and where you'd eventually like to be.

"Why do you want to stop drinking? What are your reasons for wanting to make a change?"

If drinking is causing you problems at any level, then you should feel no shame or embarrassment whatsoever in putting your hand up, asking for help and, if you need to, speaking to your GP or another professional, or confiding in a friend or family member.

If you haven't got a drinking problem and you just want to stop – hell to the yes! If you feel you *have* got a drinking problem and you're ready to make some changes you are not on your own.

It will really help to make some notes here, so grab a pen (or you can make notes on your phone) and let's go!

1. BYE BYE HANGOVERS

Let's start with an obvious one.

When did you last have a hangover? How did it make you feel physically and mentally? Was it after a big sesh and you vowed 'I'm never drinking again' (until next time) or are you finding that drinking even a small amount of booze these days means you're waking up feeling tired, groggy and snappy?

Think about the times when you've woken up in the middle of the night dying for a glass of water or reached for a leftover can of fizzy pop with your mouth feeling drier than the Sahara. Remember waking up with your heart racing as the 3 a.m. anxiety begins to grab hold. Think about when you set yourself a rule of 'just a couple' and then somehow that couple turned into a couple more – maybe not quite enough to cause you too much stress and worry but more than enough to make you feel below par, fuzzy-headed and firing on maybe just half a cylinder rather than all of them.

Hopefully this won't feel too cringy or painful, but if you can, I'd like you to remind yourself (in detail!) of how grim it can be for you and compare it to how you feel when you wake up with a clear head. Honestly, it's a no brainer.

2. HELLO BOOZE-FREE BENEFITS

Flip back to the previous section 'What do I want to be different?' (page 59). Which of the areas that we looked at where you will see improvements when you take alcohol out of the equation really spoke to you? For example, was it more energy to spend on your family, in the gym or on a hobby you love? Perhaps you want to improve your health or you need to be more clear headed at work? Maybe you are pretty sold on the idea of glowing skin and a slimmer waist – that's fine! No judgement here!

Pick your top four or five motivators, the things you are really looking forward to in a booze-free life, and write them out here. Be as specific as you like and really try to imagine what it would feel like to see the changes you want in that area.

1. _____

2. _____

3. _____

4. _____

5. _____

3. HOW DO YOU WANT TO FEEL?

Now try to picture you when you no longer want to drink. Imagine going to an event and waving away the booze without a care in the world. Think about how strong, capable and proud of yourself you will feel. It's OK if this feels a long way off, but do your very best to picture that person. If you can imagine it you are one big step closer to being it.

This is an image I want you to be able to return to if you feel yourself wavering or losing sight of what it is all for.

4. MY 'WHY' IS ...

And finally: what is your 'why'? Read back over everything you have written in this chapter so far and in Chapter 6. You might want to let it all percolate for a bit. But as soon as you feel ready, don't waste any time. Let's strike while the iron is hot and crack on while we're feeling pumped and positive!

When you are ready, distil your motivations down to a single sentence. You might need to have a few goes at this so it feels exactly right. It's a big question that deserves some thought.

I am stopping drinking because ...

_____

_____

_____

DANNY'S STORY

In my mid-thirties, I found I could only drink the way I really wanted to at home on my own. No one could have an opinion or interfere; everyone could piss off and I became happily miserable.

When I first tried to stop drinking, I decided I didn't need to associate with anyone. I armed myself with every quit-lit book on the market, I subscribed to every sobriety podcast, and with my newfound determination to never drink again I began my eight-year career as what I can only describe as a chronic, relapsing alcoholic.

By the pandemic year of 2020, my alcoholism had progressed to such a stage that each time I fell off the wagon and picked up a drink, I physically could not stop drinking. Nothing I was doing was working and I was scared. In 2020 I relapsed eight times.

I listened to the Over the Influence (OTI) podcast but they were far too positive for me. What Shaz and Ben were raving on about was not my experience of sobriety. I didn't find it joyful or magical; I found it miserable and hard. But I liked them, they made me laugh, though I never thought I would join their community. All this stuff about 'connection' was bullshit. I knew it wouldn't work for me.

Then, one night in October 2021, at six months sober, I was about to relapse again, but I did something I've never done before and I messaged the only number I had in my phone of a contact from an alcohol-free community I had previously joined, looking for validation that I would be OK going for a drink.

The contact messaged me straight back and told me a horror story about his drinking that had happened since we had last messaged each other (months before) and it stopped me in my tracks. I didn't go the pub that night. This connection had stopped me drinking.

Later that night, I joined the OTI community. I thought that while I may be cynical about yet another online sobriety group, if I was going to give this one last shot, I would make it a proper attempt, so I threw myself into the community both feet first. This time, I got to know people on Zoom calls and became familiar with their challenges and successes in sobriety, while being open and honest about mine. This all helped to put me on an unbelievable journey of self-discovery that would see me develop vulnerability, openness and self-awareness, which led to happiness, the most amazing friendships and, above all, real and lasting sobriety.

I met people from the community in real life for walks, coffees and lunches. None of these were friendships I wanted when I joined, but these 'community members' were fast becoming closer friends than any of my others, as we had that shared common goal to live alcohol-free and we spoke with each other so much.

I got to one year sober and started hosting Zoom calls myself to help other community members, which in turn helped me.

So much has changed for the better in my life that there is far too much to list. I look back at this chain of events now and can't believe where I was and how that could turn into where I am now. The way I live my life is completely the opposite of everything I used to do. Because of this, I have now not only been sober for longer than I ever have before, but I know this time it is forever.

My personality and the enthusiasm I have for life now is the real me, which is nothing like who I was in my drinking days, and this is because of community and connection. For the first time in my life, I am not happily miserable – I am happily and gratefully sober.

"With patience and determination, magic awaits you"

CHAPTER 8

Why 100 days?

Well, there are lots of reasons why I am strongly encouraging you to go all in on 100 days with no booze. Firstly, ONE HUNDRED is a wonderful number and a massive milestone to achieve. It is a decent chunk of time to get under your (possibly shrinking) belt after what might have been numerous attempts at a run up with a few trips and stumbles over the years. The confidence those three digits will give you will be immense.

As I've mentioned, I'd done thirty-day stints here and there (not always successfully but God loves a trier!) but the problem was that:

a) A month is not long enough to feel the full amazing spectrum of benefits, and

b) I was in totally the wrong mindset, always working towards drinking again. Thirty days was just long enough to prove my point that I *could* manage without booze. Then I'd dive straight back into drinking again, undoing any of the good work that would've eventually led to the magic beginning to kick in.

When you fully commit to 100 days of no alcohol without compromise, you remove so much more of the noise of the inner monologue that can rear its ugly head when you least expect it. The ridiculous arguments you find yourself having, just when you thought you were doing really well. Justifying to yourself why it would be OK to have 'just one', telling yourself 'it was never that bad' or celebrating a whole alcohol-free (AF) month with a small glass of fizz. Don't do it! Even if it wasn't that bad, remind yourself of why it will be so much better without! When you slam the door shut on booze for fourteen weeks and lock it behind you (you don't need to throw away the key, just hide it for now!), you have so much more power to silence the annoying whine of the Wine Witch and the loud grunts from the Lager Monster who, without doubt, will be knocking loudly for your attention at some point over the next few weeks.

In the years I've been sober and running the online sober community, I have yet to speak to a single person – and I mean not ONE – who has hit the triple-figure milestone of 100 days and not felt the positives and reaped the many, many benefits that come with an AF life.

And while we're on the subject, don't let the word 'sober' put you off either. I used to be a bit hesitant to use it as at first I felt embarrassed about telling others I was sober. Now, I proudly shout about it. It's a word to be embraced and it means so much more than just not being drunk!

When I started on my 100 days, I often doubted myself. I would look at people who were much further ahead on their

"Stopping drinking is like getting a load of free perks, tiny little rays of sunshine that don't cost you a penny" journey and say things like 'It's impossible', 'I wish I was where they are' and 'How on earth have they done that?'. It's so important to remember that everyone has a Day 1 and those further on in their AF adventure have been exactly where you are. So try not to feel deflated, demotivated or out of your depth. With patience and determination, magic awaits you.

And you will need these things as the positive changes I'm banging on about won't happen overnight. That's why we have to commit for the long haul. I drank for the best part of thirty years. That's three decades in which alcohol was simply a part of my life. You will not undo years of habitual drinking overnight. Or in two weeks. Those changes do come slowly, but surely. If you're removing relatively low levels of alcohol, the chances are you're going to experience the positives more quickly than someone drinking at higher levels and more regularly. If you have been drinking more and more often, you will almost certainly notice the change more acutely – but it might take longer. Oh man, it seemed to take me forever to get there but it was worth it a million times over.

I'm really hoping that your curiosity and interest in trying a life without alcohol is strong enough at this point for you to give it a serious go! If the thought of 100 days without a drink seems a bit overwhelming to you at this stage, I understand completely how you're feeling, but trust me, it's completely achievable. In the grand scheme of life, 100 days actually isn't that long at all. Let's break it down and give it some context …

According to the Office for National Statistics, the average life expectancy for a woman living in the UK in 2020–2022 was 82.6 years and 78.6 years for a man, so you're looking at an average of around 80 years.

There are approximately 29,200 days in 80 years …

… so a break of 100 days from booze in a lifetime of hopefully 80 years is just 0.34 per cent of your life – not even half a per cent! It's such a short amount of time in the grand scheme of things yet definitely long enough to put you firmly on a life-changing path. That is sort of magic if you think about it. What else can you achieve in 3.3 months that will change your life so much for the good?

This milestone of 100 days is something we very much like to celebrate in the Over the Influence (OTI) community too. A couple of years ago on the podcast, a throwaway comment was made that the Queen of Sobriety (me, apparently) should send you a handwritten OTI telegram once you hit 100 consecutive days alcohol-free. OMG. The number of emails and messages that came in were ridiculous! No joke, they were from all over the globe. Since then, I'm pretty sure that in 99.99 per cent of cases, I've managed to write to every single person in the community who has told us that they have hit their triple-figure milestone. Although, by 'telegram', I really mean a no-expense spent postcard! Regardless, these continue to get posted across the world because 100 *is* the magic number, and because it's such a boost having that positive acknowledgement that you're on the right path.

"What else can you achieve in 3 months that will change your life so much for the good?"

Stopping drinking is like getting a load of free perks, tiny little rays of sunshine that don't cost you a penny. I hope you are ready to try it, as over the next 100 days you're going to experience, see, smell and feel things that you might not have done for a very long time. The bird song is louder (and far less annoying), the colour of the flowers is so much brighter and food tastes better. I'm well aware I might sound a bit bonkers but the fact is that even the smallest amounts of alcohol can 'numb out' so much of life, messing with our hormones and our neurotransmitters, and we don't even notice this is the case until alcohol is removed completely.

CHAPTER 9

When shall
I start?

So many people ask me 'When is a good time to start?'. 'Should I put it off until I've got <insert event here> out of the way?'

I've had many, many years of bitter experience at attempting these dry spells and I can now tell you hand on heart that THERE IS NEVER A RIGHT TIME. The best time is NOW. Literally now. Don't wait any longer!

I know some people really love the idea of a significant date to mark a fresh start, such as a new month to signal new beginnings, so if this is you then fair enough. But if you're reading this on the second of the month, it's a long way off until the next one so consider starting today or tomorrow, and if that thought fills you with dread then go for this coming weekend! You get the gist ...

Though, having said that, for me, September turned out to be a brilliant month to put down the bottle and tackle the incoming Autumn with a fresh head and renewed vigour. The kids were back at school and college, home life was a tad quieter, the chaotic summer holidays fuelled by booze were over and I could focus on me and my not drinking. Fresh starts all round.

You really don't have to be at the mercy of the time of year or the social events in your diary to begin your new, exciting normal, though. With the right plan in place (more on this in a moment), you can *make* now into exactly the right time.

The fear of getting started living without booze can't be any worse than the dread recovering from drinking brings though, can it? So weigh up the scales of dread accordingly and choose the path you know is going to be better for you both mentally and physically in a million different ways. Trust me on this!

Don't wait, because the honest truth is you'll be waiting forever and as my podcast co-host, Ben, often says: 'Why wait to feel great?!' Corny with a side of cheese but it's so, so true!

You will ALWAYS have something in the diary. There is ALWAYS something going on. A friend is ALWAYS having a gathering. Kids ALWAYS have birthdays. Friday night on the sofa will ALWAYS come around. If you're looking for an excuse to drink, you'll ALWAYS find one and it's so important to turn those EXCUSES for drinking into your REASONS not to.

The chances are that if you're reading this because you're looking for a bit of inspiration and motivation to get going, then that time is *now*. What are you waiting for?

In William Porter's book *Alcohol Explained 2: Tools for a Stronger Sobriety*, he says, 'The best time to stop is now, it always has been and it always will be. You've already thrown away enough of your precious time and life being miserable because of a drug, why would you want to waste another single second on it?'

Amen, William!

ANGELA'S STORY

My drinking started to worry me in my early thirties when my children were both at primary school. I was a stay-at-home mum, my husband worked away and I was very lonely. Once the kids were in bed, I'd open the wine and sit in front of the TV until it had all gone. It felt like the only time I was ever truly happy – on my own and with a drink in my hand. The next morning, I'd be wracked with guilt, anxiety and shame. I just wanted to feel well, to be a good mum and to give my girls the life they deserved. But I didn't feel capable and I hated myself for it. Why couldn't I just be normal?

After nearly eight years of trying to quit or master moderation, the Covid-19 lockdowns arrived. They were catastrophic for my mental health and my alcohol consumption increased again. I was so isolated, now working from home with two kids, while my husband was working away for weeks on end. Every day was a wine day. When we came out of the lockdowns, my drinking slowed a little but I struggled more than ever with my mental health. Things eventually came to a head after one particularly magnificent hangover and I finally decided I was DONE with alcohol in June 2022.

This was the best thing I could have ever done for myself and my family. The accountability and support

I've received through the Over the Influence online community has changed my life. I got through the early weeks and months following the tips I'd been given by others and trusting that all the good things those who were further on in their alcohol-free (AF) adventure talked about would be coming for me. And they did!

Since then, I've had challenges with perimenopause and realised that I'm neurodivergent. The latter has been difficult to digest but I am thrilled to be where I am now – FREE! Free of shame and self-loathing, free to be me and free to follow my own path. All because I stopped drinking.

As I write this, I'm sitting among 200 cardboard boxes in my beautiful new home. After two years of being AF, we decided to become a little more financially free too. We sold our silly house in a fancy location and moved up the road into a lovely little home, which is perfect for us. Living AF has given us the courage to live a life in accordance with our hopes and dreams, rather than societal expectations. This is probably the coolest thing to ever happen to me. I've also recently handed in my notice at a job I no longer enjoy and there's lots of excitement about what will happen for me next. Now that alcohol no longer poisons the joy in my life, there's no stopping me!

CHAPTER 10

. . . .

What's the plan?

So how are you going to make a plan to support you in your alcohol-free (AF) journey? There are a few really easy, practical things you can do right now to help set yourself up for sober success over the next 100 days.

Even with the steeliest determination, nothing is ever simple and often things *don't* go to plan despite our very best intentions. Work, kids, life can absolutely get in your way but this doesn't matter because you're going to work around any stumbling blocks with positivity, clarity, strength and determination. And preparing for them in advance is the best advice I can give you at this point.

REMOVE TEMPTATION

It's a bit of an obvious one but get rid of any booze you've got in the house if you think there is even a *chance* you may be tempted or triggered to drink it. Pour any half-drunk bottles, dregs and leftovers down the sink, give away anything that's unopened or just tip it down the sink too. You'll not be needing it. (It's also quite fun and liberating to do this, in my experience!) You could also politely ask those you live with not to drink around you at home for the next few weeks while you're finding your AF feet.

Since I stopped drinking, I've always been happy to have alcohol in the house. I'm not tempted to drink it and I don't find other people drinking in the least bit triggering, but this might not be the case for you. However, even though I'm not bothered about being around booze or having it at home I have changed my rules and put boundaries in place. Previously, I'd spend hundreds of pounds stocking up on boozy supplies if we had people round. I was only ever really stocking up for myself anyway and would always buy *my* drinks of choice without even considering any AF options for those who might not be drinking. Any excuse at all, as God forbid I ever ran out! Now if we have a social gathering at home, family and friends will bring their own alcoholic drinks. They're so respectful of the fact I no longer choose to drink and they'll always bring AF options too, which is massively appreciated. Gone are the days where I'm spending my hard-earned cash on booze. It no longer serves me so I no longer choose to waste my money on it.

Think carefully about how you want this to work for you and what makes you feel more confident and comfortable. Set your own rules and boundaries from the start. Try not to worry about doing so and always remind yourself WHY you're doing this. Those who care and who genuinely want the best for you will have no problem at all respecting your choices. If your partner is reluctant to part with everything in the booze

"Don't be scared
of vocalising
how you feel"

cupboard, could you ask them to move it well out of the way – even to a friend's house – just temporarily for the first few weeks, if you think that's going to be useful for you?

Don't be scared of vocalising how you feel. Let others know this is incredibly important to you and that you'd really value and appreciate their support.

DECIDE WHAT YOU ARE
GOING TO DRINK INSTEAD

One of the first big social events I had to navigate without a glass of alcohol in my hand was my nephew's christening, when I was about six weeks in to what at that point I thought was just going to be 100 days off the booze. Previously, I'd have been straight to the bar ordering a large wine (whoever drank small or medium glasses? I always thought they were utterly pointless). This was the first time I'd ever ordered an alcohol-free drink, as I didn't want pint after pint of cola, lemonade or kids' squash. I wanted an alcohol-free alternative that would hopefully scratch an itch and taste half-decent. I asked for an alcohol-free beer and the guy behind the bar looked at me as though I'd suddenly grown a second head.

'A what?'

'An alcohol-free beer, please, whatever you've got …'

He eventually managed to locate me a warm, dusty bottle of Kaliber that I think had been there since the late 1980s. It was rank but I needed something to hold in my hand during the party and it was my only AF option that wasn't squash or fizzy pop.

However, please be reassured that the alcohol-free landscape has thankfully changed for the better. So many more people are saying no to booze now and therefore restaurants and bars often have a decent – even impressive – alcohol-free offering. Lots of cocktail bars have a section of their menu devoted to no-booze options that are just as Insta-worthy as their alcoholic counterparts. AF lager? Yes please, with a slug of lime if you don't mind or a lemonade top! AF cider with ice in the sunshine? Hits the spot. Pimped up AF G&T? Oooh, how swanky … yes, I'll have some seasonal berries in there too! Glass of fizz? Make it a chilled Nozeco and we're laughing!

In the early days, it was stuff like this that got me through. Not so much because I was hankering for the alcohol, it was more to do with wanting to feel included as an adult and have a decent choice of things to drink. However, interestingly, as I began to rack up more days free of booze, I drank them less and less. I do still enjoy an AF cocktail or gin if we're having a family celebration out at a restaurant somewhere and I'm quite partial to a non-alcoholic Martini Vibrante with ice and a slice or a can of Free Dam 0.0 lemon shandy in the sunshine in the garden, but I don't feel the need to have something in my hand that looks like a drink so much any more. It's more that these drinks taste good – better than actual alcohol AND you can still function the day after drinking them! Win win!

If Saturday night is takeaway and beer in front of the telly, you can still do that, as so many beer brands make non-alcoholic versions! Or if your thing is cooking a Sunday roast with a bottle of red on the go, you can still do that too, but instead choose an AF bottle. The choice these days is superb and it warms my cockles no end that thankfully the market is adapting to cater for people who are choosing not to drink for a million different reasons. You can now buy an AF alternative to pretty much anything you used to drink.

It must be noted, though, that AF drinks are not for everyone. Depending on your levels of drinking, you may find them triggering – be it the smell, the act of pouring a drink, the taste and the after-effects. Even though drinks classed as AF are 0.5 per cent and below, you sometimes find, particularly with the beers, that you still have a headache the morning after the night before, and that can sometimes be an unpleasant reminder of what you're trying to move away from. AF alternatives are totally your choice. I know loads of successfully sober people who've never touched them and don't really see the point, preferring to stick to fizzy water, and equally I know tons more, myself included, who say that in the early days in particular they were an absolute lifesaver during social occasions and even at home too. If you're not triggered by them then it's brilliant to have these choices to go to should you feel like it.

Funnily enough, I rarely drink AF wine, which is odd considering white and rosé used to be my first alcoholic drink of choice. I tried the AF version of one of my Spanish favourites a few years ago. But it tasted and smelt too much like the bad old days, so I never touched it again.

TWO HACKS FOR AF DRINKING

1. Think about what you like to drink that isn't booze (I don't mean just AF alternatives to alcoholic drinks) and make sure you have stocks at home. For example:

- Fancy squash

- Kombucha

- More grown-up fizzy drinks, like Sanpellegrino or Cawston Press

- Your favourite fruity or herbal teas

- A good old can of Diet Coke or other fizzy pop

- Posh hot chocolate

This is especially useful to stop you feeling 'deprived' if someone you live with is still drinking, as it gives you something to pour yourself in the evening.

2. If you are going out for dinner or to a bar, look at the drinks menu online first. Then you can order confidently when you get there, without having to ask 'What alcohol-free options do you have?'. This is useful if you think you might feel self-conscious about not drinking in the early days.

OPEN YOUR DIARY

Now, sit down with a brew, have a look at your diary and see what's coming up. If it's looking pretty clear, make the most of a few quiet weekend evenings. Staying in, doing nothing, watching TV or enjoying an early night with a book are all completely valid ways to spend your time. Particularly at the beginning.

If you've already committed to an event that you think may be difficult to navigate stone cold sober this early on, take a moment to consider your options. Is it essential you're there? Would it really matter if you were to swerve it?

If you can't, could you stay for a bit then leave? Would you feel confident on your first night out sticking with AF options? Work out what's right for you. Right now, you are doing something difficult but potentially life changing, so it's OK to prioritise that.

I can't stress this enough: it's perfectly fine for you to say 'No, thank you' to *anything* that you feel might compromise your strength or resolve. You can say no to a drink that's offered, you can decline to be part of a round (that way you're in charge of what you're drinking!), your share of a split restaurant bill doesn't have to include the wine you didn't drink and you can turn down any invitation you wish. The words 'no' and 'none' worked wonders for me in the early days. Yes, I did sometimes worry that some of my friends would think I was boring. But don't worry, this all changes. I wasn't boring – though staying on the booze carousel, repeating the same old mistakes, that was definitely boring.

MAKE SOME FUN SOBER PLANS

What does your social life look like right now? What do you enjoy doing with friends? Where do you spend most of your time socialising with others?

I'm not going to lie, if you're used to being a social butterfly, learning how to navigate sobriety can be more daunting in the beginning. Remember that you don't have to give up on socialising altogether: you can go for nice dinners or grab a coffee and cake, go to the cinema, theatre or a concert; it doesn't have to revolve around drinking. Once you remove alcohol – and again, this comes over time – you discover exactly how and where you want to spend your social time. And more often than not, it's NOT in a boozy bar or on a pub crawl!

This is the perfect time to think about booking in some early morning weekend activities (whatever 'early' means for you!). I'm not talking about climbing mountains at sunrise or training for an ultra-marathon in the desert (although don't let me stand in your way if that's what you want!). Start off with something small and achievable that's going to make you feel good at the same time too.

Not been to the gym in a while? See if there's a Saturday morning class you could try. Fancy catching up with a friend? Suggest going for a Sunday morning walk followed by breakfast or brunch. Kids need entertaining? Take them swimming! Or find out where your local parkrun is taking place and get yourself there at 9 a.m. on a Saturday (you don't even have to

"If you've got a few nice things in the diary that don't revolve around booze, you're much less likely to feel like you're missing out" run the 5km route, you can just walk it). These events across the UK (and around the world) are friendly, fun and free, and a brilliant activity to try in your early days. (Side note: I ended up running the London Marathon about four years after my first ever parkrun. Before that, I couldn't even run a bath. I factored this superb Saturday morning event into my initial three-month plan regularly and, to everyone's surprise, absolutely loved it.)

It's fine if running isn't at all your thing (although, who knows what you might learn about yourself now you're ditching the booze …!). The point is, if you've got something to get up for on your weekend mornings, you're far less likely to drink the night before and cry off because you've already made yourself accountable. And if you've got a few nice things in the diary that don't revolve around booze – even if it's just a date with a Netflix series you've been saving – you're much less likely to feel like you're missing out.

ASSEMBLE YOUR CHEER SQUAD

At the very least, think of a few people who you can tell about your resolution to ditch the booze and how they might be able to support you. There's more about what and how you tell people coming up (page 127), but if you know someone who has been there and done it, they will most likely be thrilled for you and could be a useful person to speak to early on.

If you have friends and family who rarely if ever drink, this is a good time to plan a meet up.

A really great way of navigating potentially tricky social situations and also working out which friends are on your side is to make suggestions of new things to do and places to go. Planning activities during the daytime is hugely helpful in the early days. Swap a wine and takeaway night in for a walk and takeout coffee afternoon out. Go somewhere you've never been before and invite your friends along. You'll find that friends want to spend time with you and it doesn't always have to involve drinking. You may find that some love the idea of activities that don't revolve around late nights and bars.

TAKE A PHOTO

Now please don't laugh at this one … but you need to take a Day 1 photo! It's probably going to make you cringe and admittedly it might not be your best look BUT what you're then going to do is take another in a couple of weeks time and put the two side by side. If it makes you feel any better, I look absolutely terrible on my Day 1 selfie. You can almost smell the hangover and taste the vodka in the photo! It's SO bad. My skin is grey with red blotches, one of my eyes is higher than the other, my nose is wonky, my lips are thin and I just look really sad. This is such a brilliant exercise to do because even though you might not be *feeling* great straight away you will absolutely begin to *see* the little magical effects that not drinking is already having even after just a couple of weeks.

MILESTONES

A great way to keep you on track is to make sure that you consciously acknowledge along the way that you're doing something amazing and celebrate those mini milestones. It might be the first time in a very long time you've managed a whole week or a fortnight without alcohol. So celebrate with cake! One month alcohol-free? Buy a new book! Halfway through your 100 days? That's worthy of a pamper day or a ticket to a gig!

Self-care is key, so as part of your personalised plan, factor in some lovely stuff just for you over the coming weeks that's going to bring you a little bit of joy. If those thoughts of reward involve 'just the one', bat them away immediately. There are so many other ways you can spoil yourself that don't involve booze. Most of mine were food and sugar based in those first three months (and continue to be so!). Think about what you'd like to mark these occasions now, so you have something in your mind to look forward to.

You are going to feel so different at thirty days to how you felt after one week sober. You'll be a whole new person after seventy days, compared to who you were after twenty-one. I'm a big advocate of tracking your progress and giving yourself the highly deserved pats on the back, so on page 247, you'll find a template for a milestone tracker to help make sure you celebrate all those wins.

CONSIDER KEEPING A DIARY

If you already love a bit of journalling, you're probably planning to do this already. But even if the thought of writing your feelings down makes your toes curl, don't dismiss it out of hand, as documenting your feelings and observations from the beginning is another huge motivation to keep you on track during the 100 days. You can find your own way to do this.

Earlier in the book, I asked you to note how drinking made you feel, especially in the days afterwards. Another great exercise to do now is to keep a record of how you're feeling *without* the booze. You can do this as your first task of the day or at the end of the day as a reflection exercise. Compare how you're feeling now to how you felt while drinking. The chances are you're going to be blown away by the difference, particularly as the number of days since your last drink ticks ups. Also take time to note what you were like socially when you were on the pop compared to going out now and *not* drinking.

•   •   •

There is just one hard and fast rule to follow over the next 100 days – don't drink. Your AF journey is going to be different to mine and to that of the next person giving it a go. If all you're managing to do at the moment is not drink, you're winning. The key here, as I hope you've gathered from this section, is to be proactive and try to figure out what is going to work for you. What are your triggers going to be and what plan do you need to have in place so you can swerve the bear traps? You might have to adjust and tweak as you go along but that's OK. You'll figure it out. Keep going back to your 'why'.

I bought myself a calendar to hang on the office wall at work and each day I didn't drink I crossed it off with a big red 'X'. I absolutely loved this daily visual reminder of the positive steps I was taking. I unfollowed all the 'mummy drinking culture' accounts on social media and replaced them with sobriety accounts. I bought every quit-lit book under the sun (page 245) to make sure I could arm myself with the right tools when and where needed. I listened to sober podcasts for the same reasons. I told anyone who'd listen what I was doing to make myself accountable and I began to blog my journey from Day 1. I put absolutely all my efforts into NOT drinking, gave it 100 per cent, no half-arsed measures and just full-on slammed the door shut on alcohol for what was only going to be a three-month break to see what might happen.

So get your own plan in place – and really go for it. Don't worry right now if you will drink again or not. The more prepared you are, the better chance of success. Know that it's completely normal to feel thoroughly pissed off in the first couple of weeks! But it's building up the little early wins that will eventually get you there, I promise. Don't think of it as what you're giving up or missing out on. Reframe it and know that it's about everything you're going to gain.

WHAT CAN I EXPECT IN THE
FIRST THIRTY-ISH DAYS?

You might sail through the first few weeks excited by the novelty of your plan and new routine … and then find yourself bored and listless after three weeks.

You could plod through well enough, taking each day as it comes … and then the football season starts and watching a match in the pub without a pint feels wrong and disappointing.

You might really struggle to know what to do with yourself to start with … then get a big burst of motivation when you realise that you feel and look great … and then begin to dread your first big sober social event.

The point is, we are all different. As I have said before, no two people's journeys to the magic 100 are going to be the same. But it is in these early days that you sow those little magical seeds of hope. It takes time and it takes patience, as you can't undo decades of drinking in just a couple of weeks. But every day you nail being alcohol-free is a massive win and it's all part of the life-changing magic of quitting alcohol. Every time you navigate doing something without booze that previously you would have definitely had a drink in your hand for, it's like adding a little bit of superpower into your invisible AF rucksack, making you stronger and better able to tackle the next challenge, then the next one and the one after that.

I *did not* feel the life-changing magic of sobriety in my first few alcohol-free weeks. I hope this doesn't happen to you but I want you to be prepared in case it does, so you recognise what's going on, grit your teeth, suck it up and stick with it!

My Day 1 was always going to be a shitshow because I knew I had a 'start date' and I was going to go out with a bang. If I wasn't drinking for 100 days, I sure as hell was going to drink as much as I could on my 'final' day of boozing! The hangover I had the following day was proof I'd completed what I'd set out to do with knobs on – and that I was doing exactly what I needed to be doing, as this relationship with booze had gone on quite long enough. Don't do what I did. You're far better off tipping the booze down the sink rather than down your neck. It's pointless and just not worth it!

The first four weeks continued to be absolutely shite. Imagine the biggest turd emoji possible, double it, and that gives you an idea of my mentality. I was tired, angry, agitated and bored. I felt like I was missing out. I hated not knowing how to switch off on a Friday night. I hated the perceived boredom. I hated not having a buzz. I assumed that everyone else was having fun without me and I hated the fact that this miserable nonsense was going to continue for a whole three months. At this point, I 'knew' I was going to return to drinking on 1 December but still, THREE MONTHS?! What was the point?

I reluctantly, resentfully, sucked it up, put a plan in place, pushed through the frustration and stuck to it ... And very slowly, day by day, my life began to change for the better, even if I didn't notice it immediately at the time.

One problem I had to begin with was that I couldn't fathom for the life of me how anyone could be SO exhausted by *not* drinking, especially as I was no longer living in the fog of a hangover. I was baffled and a bit pissed off that stopping drinking hadn't instantly made me feel better, and I actually began to think that something was seriously wrong with me. I kept googling 'full body health check', 'health MOT for women over 40' and 'I've stopped drinking, I still feel like shit, what the fuck's wrong with me?' I'd never known exhaustion like it. I'd come home from work and just sleep on the sofa. I could nod off at two in the afternoon and wake up there in the dark at two in the morning! No matter how much I slept I just couldn't shake the tiredness and I came very close to booking an appointment with my GP followed by a £600 private health check. In the end, neither was necessary. My knackered middle-aged body was simply resetting after years of having to cope with the alcohol.

When I got to around three months in, it all changed. The fog began to lift and it was like the brightest light being switched back on. Hallelujah! But that is telling, isn't it? That it took my body three whole months to wean itself off this drug I had been merrily putting into it for decades and get over the shock that I was no longer drinking.

The positive changes did start making themselves known earlier, though. They were small to start with, but significant enough for me to begin feeling good. Not brilliant, not overnight, but I soon realised that I felt considerably better than I did.

I was instantly more productive. There's no doubt that removing alcohol can leave a hole. Cooking while having a wine in the kitchen, drinking with dinner, sitting down and having a couple to relax because you've 'earned' it when the kids have gone to bed, socialising at weekends. Initially, I just felt annoyed about what I couldn't have. But soon enough, I saw that when you remove booze – however much you drink – there's a gap to fill. You have so much more time, your motivation levels are not being hijacked by what you drank and it's amazing just how much you can get done!

Also, prior to stopping drinking, I had aches and pains that were obviously heavily influenced by what I had drunk. I used to get an acid-type burning in my chest, I'd have throbs and aches in places I shouldn't and, after a particularly boozy do, I'd have pains and bruises that I couldn't account for, caused by falling over and into things while sloshed. Of course, I couldn't feel them at the time as the alcohol was an anaesthetic. As if by magic, all this stopped when I removed the alcohol.

One more warning about the early days – I think you're probably going to cry. Chances are you're not going to know why either, but if you've been drinking heavily for many, many years, the tears and emotions can hit you from nowhere. With me, it was often a mixture of relief and regret. Relief I'd finally stopped putting booze first at the top of a very long list of priorities and regret that I didn't stop drinking sooner. Couple the crashing waves of emotion with crippling tiredness and it can leave you wondering *why* the hell you're doing this, never mind asking yourself how!

But you are. You can and you will! If I can get though all of this, committed and obsessive drinker that I was, and come out the other side not missing alcohol in the slightest, then you can too.

SOCIALISING

If the thought of socialising without booze at first seems too much, that is fine. As discussed earlier, you can say no (page 100). But if you've got an important event already in the diary, the only way to find out what it's going to be like sober is to flippin' do it!

Think about what you are going to drink instead. Have an idea of when you want to leave. If it's no fun at all, well, you can get through a few hours, can't you? It's not going to last for ever. And if it's surprisingly better than you thought it would be – winner! Yes, it's going to feel different, but so are you when you've nailed it and woken up the next day feeling as proud as (AF) punch!

Nothing in your life will change if you keep repeating the same behaviours. Do it differently and be brave. Just try it.

However, as a caveat to all this, in these early days, it is essential to stick with the people that want this to stick for you. I've already said it, but you can't tackle this half-arsed – and half-arsed cheerleaders aren't going to work either. Your full arse is required at all times, as is that of your circle. (Yes, I am going to leave you with that mental image and move right on!) There's more to come on what to say to nosy people and naysayers (a.k.a. people secretly worried about their own drinking), but at the beginning, if you think such people are likely to put you off your stride, just dodge them.

How many times in the past have you said, 'Oh, go on then!' to someone who's offered you a drink, despite you having told them that you're currently trying to knock it on the head? Why do we do that? (Why do they do that?!) Because sometimes it's just the easiest thing to do. There's zero effort required on your part and it puts an end to any conversations and questions you can't be arsed with.

Let's just acknowledge that for some of us, it can feel awkward, uncomfortable and confronting to say no to something that's so hugely ingrained in society and an accepted and celebrated part of everyday life. It's especially hard if, like I was, you're normally the first one to yell 'YES! And make it a large one!'. And this gets old and tiring where you want to change but you keep running up against obstacles. Start by using the words 'No, thank you' and NOT 'No, sorry'. Make no apology for it and say it with a smile! 'No' is such a simple word but one so many of us struggle to say when it comes to alcohol, both to ourselves and to others.

The more I said no to alcohol the stronger I got and the more I began to feel proud and confident in my decisions.

TRIGGERS

Triggers can be problematic in the first few weeks of your 100 days, although not necessarily for everyone. Again, this varies massively, depending on the type of drinker you are and how much and how often you drank.

A trigger is anything that makes you want to slip back into old behaviours and drink. They are things that set off the craving for a drink, be it for your usual chilled glass of wine with dinner, a beer in the sunshine or a four-day bank holiday binge. Triggers can come in the form of people, places, days of the week, routine, mood and even the weather! So, as you gingerly make your way through your first thirty days of sobriety, let's look at identifying your potential triggers, and how you can anticipate and avoid them.

- **You want to drink because you've had a bad week at work.** If you choose not to, you can tackle whatever stresses you're dealing with head-on with a clear mind and much more focus. Work has taken up enough of your energy this week. Do you really want to sacrifice feeling good this weekend *and* your good intentions to it as well by opening that bottle just because you're annoyed about what happened at work? What else can you do to make you feel less stressed?

- **You want to drink because the kids are being dicks.** Kids will always be dicks at some point (they do grow up though and become less hard work. Sort of!) but they need parents who are present and supportive not pissed and disconnected. Can you get someone to step in for an hour or so, so you can get some timeout to go

for a coffee or a gym session, or do something else you
enjoy by yourself?

- **You want to drink because everyone else is.** See this
chapter, page 112 on socialising and revisit your fun
sober plans from page 101. This isn't about everyone
else. This is about you. Plus I'm willing to bet that at
least some of those people with a drink in their hand
right now are going to feel panicked, gross and/or
regretful tomorrow. They are probably questioning
their drinking but haven't yet got to the amazing place
you have yet, where you are actually doing something
about it.

- **You want to drink because you always do when it's
Christmas/your birthday/the sport is on/it's Friday.**
Here's another of those motivational clichés for you: if
you don't change anything, nothing changes. And we're
here because you want things to be different from now
on, right? Don't focus on what you are choosing not to
do, but what you can do instead. To break those habits,
make new ones. Like a cracking festive mocktail that
becomes a part of your family tradition. A new birthday
ritual, like getting up to see the sun rise.

If you need to, go back to your 'why'. Take each trigger and find
a way to dismantle it or avoid it until it begins to lose its power
over you. Keep reminding yourself why you are doing this. Turn
your excuses for drinking into your reasons not to.

The biggest triggers I had to navigate during my first year of sobriety were Friday nights and sunny days.

Friday nights signalled switching off, the start of the weekend and me, me, me time after a busy working week. They were also my Massive Green Light for earlier and increased drinking.

Years ago, when my boozing was at its absolute peak and yet I still didn't think I had an 'issue', I would leave work and head to a local spinning class – an hour of cycling on a stationary bike accompanied by banging tunes and intermittent grunts of pain. I'd then drive home, sweaty and smug, feeling chuffed that I'd started my weekend in such a wholesome and healthy way.

I'd walk through the front door at home and head to the fridge to 'celebrate' my achievement by pouring two double raspberry vodkas, which I'd take upstairs with me to the bath, where I could enjoy them in peace and no one would notice I'd already had a couple by the time it came to opening my Friday night wine. 'Treating' myself to alcohol as a reward for exercising was utterly bonkers, but it was a Friday and that's all the justification I needed.

The void on a Friday night was vast when I first stopped. It felt weird and I didn't know what to do. For the first few Fridays, I refused any social invites. I knew I'd be tempted to drink and in the early days, I didn't feel strong enough to say no if alcohol was offered or if any pressure was put on me to 'just have one'.

I started to plan an activity for Saturday morning. That's when I began going to parkrun. I'd always fancied it but had been all talk and no action – or all hangover, no action. I took the kids along too and this proved a great way of distracting myself from wanting to drink on a Friday night. No way would I have had the motivation to get up early on a Saturday if I'd chosen to drink the night before. There is nothing quite like the feeling of waking up the morning after the night before when you've chosen not to drink! It might feel tough getting through that Friday, but the Saturday morning smugness proved a great reward!

My other huge trigger was glorious sunny days. I actually cried the first time the sun came out for a decent stint because I was so frustrated I 'couldn't' drink and socialise in the sunshine. Sunshine to me has always meant drinking in the garden, outside bars and pubs, at festivals and outdoor community events. I could not cope with the thought of being in the sunshine and not drinking my favourite rosé wine. So I had to put a plan in place that didn't mean jeopardising all the hard work that had got me to this point.

Of course, I could still enjoy my garden in the sunshine so I took myself off to the garden centre to buy some colourful plants and flowers, and turned a small part of our outdoor space into my little Coffee Corner. Who knew you could sit in your garden without wine and actually drink other things?!

If on those Friday nights I'd have simply continued to sit on the settee just without the wine, I'd have caved. I had to acknowledge that it was going to feel different and I was only going to rack up another AF day by doing something positive about it.

If I'd have chosen to simply sit in my garden sulking in the sunshine without a drink in my hand, I'd have continued to feel like I was missing out. So I filled the gaps and filled my pots and flower beds with the brightest colours and the prettiest blooms!

It was about doing something different. It was about identifying the trigger, noting how it made me feel and then doing something constructive to fill the wine-glass-shaped gap with something useful and productive.

We talked a bit about emotional triggers previously (page 113) – when you have been using alcohol to make yourself feel better. But often, triggers are part of your daily routine. What are your triggers now? What parts of your day or week might make you feel like you 'need' a drink? For example:

- Being around certain people and situations.
- A visit to your local pub or restaurant.
- Driving past the supermarket or wine shop on the way home from work.
- A hobby or pastime that usually finishes up in the pub, like a pint after a country walk or a game of football.

If you become aware of what your triggers are you can work around them, change your routine and do things a little bit differently. It might just be a case of deciding not to go past your regular local shop. It might be avoiding your usual local haunts for the time being. It could be planning to do

"You will become stronger and the pull of alcohol will grow much weaker" something with supportive friends or family that's not centred around alcohol during the times you'd normally have a drink. These small adjustments to your day can have a huge effect on your desire to drink and ultimately set you up for mega AF success!

Speaking from personal experience, I can reassure you that early triggers do fade once you've found ways of navigating them and learning how to deal with the urges or cravings they can create. While it may sometimes feel like it takes all of your effort and energy to not pop a bottle of nice red in the supermarket trolley or allow your feet to take you right through the door of your favourite pub, this is not forever. One day, you'll walk straight past Sainsbury's wine aisle without even noticing it, or find yourself propping up the bar completely content with the 0.0 per cent Guinness in your hand.

GLIMMERS

During your first thirty days I urge you to start looking for the glimmers. They are sort of the opposite of triggers because they spur you on rather than threatening to throw you off track. Glimmers are the little micro-moments of joy that can go unnoticed, especially when you're still drinking. Drinking dulls the senses, but when it's removed those senses are then given space to awaken and breathe.

For every single day you choose not to drink I can guarantee you will find something good in it. The more distance you put between yourself and your Day 1 the more glimmers you will see and the closer you will get to living a magical life where alcohol becomes nothing more than a distant memory.

If you find yourself walking down the road with a new spring in your step, take note.

If you realise you are singing happily along to the radio while cooking, enjoy the moment and turn up the volume!

If you try something new you wouldn't have done before and really enjoy it, send someone who is supporting you a message to tell them about it.

These moments add up. They show you that you are on the right track and doing well. You just need to make the effort to consciously notice them. They are an important motivator that will help carry you to that crucial 100 days without alcohol – official life-changing territory.

The way you feel about alcohol will change. The way you socialise will change. You will become stronger and the pull of alcohol will grow much weaker. The positives of living a sober life will begin to outweigh the perceived negatives and the scales will begin to tip.

Search for the glimmers. You won't have to look too far.

SLEEP

A quick heads up here: sleeping like a baby might not happen overnight, so bear this in mind and try not to feel too frustrated if this is the case for you.

"Take it one day at a time and have the self-belief that you can do this. You've got this!"

Waking up feeling fresh and ready to go really *is* one of the great feelings in life and it will come for you, but if you've been drinking regularly for a while, it's highly unlikely your mind and body will repair overnight and return to full factory settings in the first week.

So if, all of a sudden, you find yourself needing a nanna nap on the settee in front of the telly at the weekend, have one. If you can't stop yawning and an early night is calling, go to bed with a book and a (decaf) brew. It's one thing wasting a day in bed if you're recovering from a hangover but quite another if you're allowing your body to rest and reset because you've finally removed the stuff that was causing you issues in the first place.

Improved sleep is also very much tied in with what you might choose to do with your time to fill those gaps where previously you'd have been drinking. Getting outdoors is such a huge benefit. It's free, it's good for you and a huge dose of fresh air helps massively with sleep. It is so much more satisfying, both mentally and physically, when you go to bed feeling naturally tired rather than ruined because of drinking.

Sleeping with a belly full of booze can be fitful, erratic and disturbed. Sleeping after not drinking eventually becomes deep, restorative and nothing short of glorious. You'll begin to swap late nights and broken sleep for a wonderful eight hours of uninterrupted slumber! It comes, and when it does it's nothing short of bloody magical!

How often do we tell ourselves that we need a drink to help us sleep at night? It's yet another myth and if you want to read more about the effect even a small amount of alcohol can have on your sleep and the science behind it, I recommend William Porter's book, *Alcohol Explained* (see page 245 for more recommendations too).

• • •

I have heard so many Over the Influence community members say that they questioned their sobriety during this first thirty-day time frame. You are not alone if this is you. My podcast co-host, Ben, and I have very handily named this period the 'The Shit Zone' as, simply put, it can be overwhelmingly shit! That first hurdle is tough for many people, there's no denying it.

Belief is so important. Do not underestimate your strength and your capabilities. You're harnessing a superpower you probably didn't know you were hiding and the longer you go at this the stronger you will get. You will not feel the same on Day 10 as you did on Day 1. By Day 31 you will have a month's worth of AF days bagged. Your confidence will be growing and you'll be feeling more resilient. You might even be starting to feel excited as you head into your second month!

Some changes will be toe-curlingly uncomfortable, others will bring you nothing but increased self-esteem and pride. But the more distance you begin to put between you and Day 1, the stronger you'll get, the better you will feel and the more motivated you will be to hit the magic number of 100 days.

Drinking can be an utter recurring nightmare, but if you work out how the hell you're going to do this, then your dreams

"Each day you choose not to drink is a win"

will, with patience and a lot of hard work, begin to come true, revealing the true you. I am living proof that this will happen. You just have to take it one day at a time and have the self-belief that you can do this. You've got this!

Those who are further on in this journey can be vital sources of motivation and inspiration. For example, one of my original inspirations early on in my 100-days sobriety was the alcohol-free guru and all-round sober legend Andy Ramage. At the time, he was where I am now, and yet back then, it blew my mind that people could be five months, twelve months, two years or five years sober. How? What was this mystical sorcery?! It didn't seem possible.

But it is. It truly is! If you're feeling tired, sleep. If you want the cake, eat it. If you don't want to socialise, say no. Do whatever you need to do, for you. Each day you choose not to drink is a win. Even if all you do for that day is not drink, you're winning. You've nothing to lose and absolutely everything to gain.

CHAPTER 11

What do I tell people?

For many of us, a good chunk of the fear and worry about stopping drinking comes from how much importance we place on what others think of our decision to do so.

I hope that you have a group of supportive friends – perhaps some of whom have already decided life is more magic when it's booze-free, or who can simply take or leave it – but the reality is that if you have previously been known for your 'Where's the party?' or 'One more for the road!' attitude to life, you have likely collected a group around you who are the same. Or who may simply find it difficult initially to adjust to the new booze-free you.

There is also a fear of judgement as to what people may assume about why you stopped drinking. *What if they think I've got a problem? What if I HAVE got a problem?*

Or worry as to how best to handle the transition to a sober you in a social setting. *How do I tell people I'm not drinking next weekend? How do I say no to a drink? What if I'm offered one and I don't know how to say no?*

The list of worries can be endless in those early days, but really, when you cut through the noise and focus on what you want and where you are trying to get to on your booze-free journey, it all starts to get much easier.

Remember, this is about you. No one else.

'WHY AREN'T YOU DRINKING?'

It's always good to have a few stock answers up your sleeve and ready to go when you're cornered with your lime and lemonade or your 0.0 bottle of lager while you're out, just in case you're asked a curveball question out of the blue that might leave you flustered, a bit stuck for words and facing a situation where it could seem easier to agree to a drink rather than stay super-strong and stick to your guns. An answer that feels comfortable and easy for the particular situation you find yourself in. That allows you, if necessary, to deflect any attention that makes you feel awkward. Particularly if you're still navigating those tricky early days.

How much information about yourself are you willing to share? Who's asking the question? Why are they asking the question? Is it just out of sheer bloody nosiness? Genuine curiosity? Are they trying to imply you're a prize prick for trying sobriety? Or do they genuinely care about you and want to know how you are?

YOU DON'T OWE ANYONE ANYTHING!

You are on a journey of self-discovery, to see what lies in the sunlit uplands free from hangovers and post-drinking lethargy.

"Remember, this is about you and no one else"

If you don't fancy getting into it, though, particularly when you are still getting used to the idea yourself, then you are under no obligation to do so.

If you don't want to be quizzed by a casual acquaintance, colleague or stranger when you turn down a drink at a gathering or work event, then don't feel like you have to explain your 100 days alcohol-free journey, unless you want to. In these scenarios, you might prefer to deflect with a simple answer to quickly move the conversation on. For example:

- I am taking some medication and drinking is not recommended.
- I have a blood test tomorrow and I can't drink before it.
- I'm doing an alcohol-free challenge for charity.
- I'm just taking a break for a few weeks.
- I'm training for a half-marathon/sponsored bike ride/to become a chess grandmaster and I need to be on my A-game.

And if you want to avoid questions or comments altogether, a pimped-up tonic water in a fishbowl glass looks no different to a G&T or pour your alcohol-free (AF) beer into a glass, no one will even know. Most people are far more concerned with themselves anyway and will likely not notice.

IF YOU DO WANT TO SHARE

It's really quite empowering to be able to confidently tell people that you're done with drinking and that you just feel better without it. Who can argue with doing something that makes you feel good and, over time, improves every single aspect of your life in so many positive ways?

But if you're not at that point yet, that's fine. You don't have to stand on a chair and deliver a speech about how you are renouncing alcohol *FOR GOOD!* I just said I was doing a three month 'reset' (I still had every intention of going back to boozing at this point!) and I was determined to complete my personal alcohol-free challenge. Yes, I still got the 'just have one' and the 'you've done a month so you might as well celebrate with a drink' comments but I was able to bat them off with a firm: 'No! I'm on a challenge!'

You could simply say that you are bored with drinking, that you are sick of hangovers, that you feel SO MUCH better without it. That it's just something you're trying – but you are definitely going to stick to it for a bit. Whatever works for you. You don't need to share *War and Peace*, just tell them whatever you're happy with and keep it short and sweet!

Just make sure you have a firm follow-up 'NO, really' practised and ready to go in your head, in response to anyone who persists in offering you 'just a half! A small one!'.

"Alcohol wasn't
the magic elixir
I believed it was"

ASKING FOR SUPPORT FROM
YOUR NEAREST AND DEAREST

We are all different, as are our friends and family. I think, in general, that the more open you are with those closest to you, the easier it can be. Unless there is someone in your immediate family whose problematic relationship with alcohol is likely to affect your commitment and resolve over the next 100 days, you don't need to dance around it, hide it or think of excuses. You can just be yourself, except without alcohol. It's your shout but I'd encourage you to share with those you trust that you've set yourself a personal challenge not to drink for the next 100 days. If there is something specific they can do to help you, then ask them. They may even decide to join you. As a drinker, I used to believe alcohol was the magic potion that cemented the best of friendships and that it brought glamour, sparkle and fun to socialising. I believed alcohol made conversations more interesting and that it made evenings at home more enjoyable. But as a non-drinker, I began to learn that alcohol wasn't the magic elixir I believed it was. It was in fact a pretty weak glue that held friendships together because once it was removed, some quickly fell apart. I began to learn that alcohol distorted conversations and made them repetitive. Without booze comes listening and concentration when chatting with friends, not gossiping and distraction. It meant conversations became deeper and more interesting.

DEALING WITH NEGATIVE REACTIONS

It is really, really hard to remain motivated in the early days if some of your social circle imply that you're as dull as ditch water for not wanting to drink alcohol. You might even *feel* as dull as ditch water at first if it's a big break from the norm for you, as it's likely to be hugely out of your comfort zone. But do not worry because these initial feelings won't last for long.

For the record, you are absolutely NOT boring for wanting to make a change – a change that a lot of people aren't even brave enough to *consider*, never mind action. It's a Big Deal. YOU'RE a Big Deal. In fact, you're embarking on one of the most magical and exciting adventures of your life, even if it doesn't feel like it yet! How can that possibly be boring? Staying the same forever is boring. Staying the same when it's not working for you is even more boring still.

What I found was that in 99.9 per cent of cases, any negative reactions I got came from heavy drinkers. And I would take a guess that a lot of those people who feel the need to say something dismissive or disparaging to people working on giving up drinking are – just occasionally or quite often – worried about their own alcohol consumption. 'Who on God's earth would CHOOSE to stop drinking?' they'll boom, while inside they are quietly thinking, 'Oh God, should *I* stop drinking? Why is this person confident enough to give it a shot but I don't feel I can?'. I've yet to be told to 'just have one' or encouraged to drink by someone who is teetotal or who can take it or leave it.

"You're a Big Deal.
In fact, you're
embarking
on one of the
most magical
and exciting
adventures of
your life"

I can 100 per cent say this with total conviction because I too was once one of those boozers who would often slate people who chose not to drink and mock them with the line 'I don't trust people who don't drink!'. What a truly awful thing to say! Some of my closest friends now are non-drinkers and I'd trust them with my life. Turns out I only ever said it to fellow drinkers in a weary attempt to justify my ever-increasing consumption and make myself feel marginally better for being a drunken knob.

It's bonkers that you choosing not to drink can make other people feel uncomfortable. But that's not for you to worry about (though easier said than done, I realise!). The further you go with this, the more you'll understand that it's not and never was your sobriety that's the problem; it's more the case that you NOT drinking can shine a light on others and for some, this can be an uncomfortable position to be in, as not everyone is as strong as you in admitting to themselves that they have been drinking more than they wanted to.

But, while it might not be the case for all, the sad and hard reality may be that stopping drinking might cost you one or two friendships along the way, though hopefully just temporarily. There may also be times when you feel left out if everyone is out on the town and it's not where you want to be. It will all work itself out in the end, but you may just at times need to strap yourself in, buckle up and prepare yourself for a bumpy and turbulent ride!

One more thing I found particularly unhelpful when I told people I wasn't drinking, was that alongside the inevitable quizzing and curiosity, some people would mutter something about how they only drink at weekends and ask why the hell couldn't I just moderate my intake. No shit, Sherlock! Do you not think I've tried that old chestnut around a million times over the last decade?

However, eventually, I realised that every time I successfully navigated yet another social occasion with the questioning and prying, I tightened up my spiel, believed in myself a little more when I said 'I don't drink' or 'I am not drinking at the moment', and it made me just that little bit stronger for the next time and added to my determination to keep going.

* * *

Remember, drinking in a crowd is seemingly all fun and games at the time. Fast forward to the morning and days after and you're well and truly on your own! No one is coming to save you and only you can take that leap off the hangover hamster wheel of hell. This is why it's SO important to put yourself front, middle and centre without apology and stay super strong in your resolve. Your future self is already thanking you for it and your past self is kicking your ass and asking why on earth you didn't do this sooner!

Being totally honest, over the years, I have found myself crying about some friendship group and social life changes that I've experienced since I decided to stop drinking. There have been times when I've felt left out, laughed at, talked about and ignored. It can be a bitter pill to swallow when you realise you've not been invited to something and you find out all about it on social media a few days later. But I had to repeatedly remind myself who I was doing this for. Me. No one else, just me.

But equally, I've also cried tears of total joy and happiness when friends have embraced my sobriety with me and celebrated the fact I no longer choose to drink. I unlocked aspects of my life that were to be the most exciting I've ever experienced, like spending quality time with my family and being able to recall all the details – something I hadn't considered when I was in the midst of booze. This was another magical surprise I could not have predicted.

I was often surprised that when I shared my alcohol-free journey, though some were predictably negative, other people were immediately full of words of encouragement and a genuine wish for me to succeed. Then, the longer I went and the stronger I got in sobriety, the more people felt they could open up to me about their own drinking and confide in me about their worries – something which I'm SO passionate about and what in many ways inspired me to write this book. That sort of reaction never occurred to me on that horrible, hungover Day 1 of not drinking. So, remember, at first they'll ask you WHY you're doing it and further down the line they may well be asking you HOW you're doing it.

HELEN'S STORY

My drinking was like Russian roulette – some nights I would stay in control, others I'd end up doing things I'd regret. I thought alcohol helped me cope with my stressful job. When my mum and a close friend both suddenly got sick with cancer and died, I used it to blot out the feelings. I'm a doctor and I felt so hypocritical telling patients to drink less. I felt deeply ashamed that I hadn't been able to 'control' alcohol and I kept it quiet when I eventually decided to stop.

My sleep was better, my face less bloated, my blood pressure and resting heart rate reduced. I felt much more calm without alcohol and I was coping much better with stress. Though even after a few years alcohol-free, I was very nervous talking about it in work because I thought an alcohol problem might be seen as unprofessional. I didn't have any friends who were sober.

When I discovered Over the Influence, my eyes suddenly opened to a world where being sober was a positive lifestyle choice, fun things happened and there were so many others doing the same thing. It was amazing. It was the first time I'd thought being alcohol-free was something to be proud of. I began to connect and share my story. The more I talked about being sober, the easier it got.

A lightbulb moment for me was listening to a podcast episode talking about shame. I realised I HAD been ashamed but I didn't need to be.

I wrote an article for my professional journal about going sober. I got amazing feedback; people mentioned it at conferences and I got emails from fellow doctors. It was such a good feeling.

I'm training for a marathon, I'm 20kg lighter, my life is so full and active. I feel like I am my true, authentic vulnerable self, living my best life.

I now see that not drinking is a huge positive and that it doesn't matter how much you drink ... if it's too much for you, then it's too much.

I'm feeling excited about what's next for me. I have found so many changes came about when I stopped drinking alcohol. I'm hoping to successfully run that marathon this year and I just love that I have options to do anything. I'm loving getting more and more authentic and more the real me as time goes on.

CHAPTER 12

What else might help me?

So you have committed to the 100 days. You have your tailor-made plan in place and you are plodding – or skipping, if you are nothing like me at all! – through the first few weeks, carefully bodyswerving any triggers. What other tools can you add to your sober kit?

ACCOUNTABILITY

We've talked a bit about what you might tell people about the change you are making to your relationship with alcohol, but what I've not yet touched on is the importance of accountability.

As we've discussed in the previous chapter, you might not feel brave enough just yet to share publicly that you're taking a break from the booze; I absolutely understand that putting yourself out there can make you feel overwhelmed and exposed. But there is so much value in finding ways to make yourself accountable.

Personally, I was very vocal about my decision to remove booze from Day 1, with my nearest and dearest and across my social media too. I knew that by doing so it would increase my accountability levels massively and keep me on track. I also knew some people would think it was a ridiculous idea and wouldn't hesitate to tell me I couldn't do it, which in itself would motivate me. Because I'm bloody-minded and as stubborn as an ox when it comes to doubters, I absolutely WILL do that thing you've just told me I can't!

What helped me massively on one of the occasions I gave up for a full month – a stepping stone on the road to my 100 days – was signing up to the official Macmillan Cancer Support challenge and raising a few quid in the process. As well as supporting a good cause, it was the public accountability that was key. Sharing what I was doing with family and friends in group chats and on social media meant I was less likely to let people down and scupper my plans in the tricky early days of a dry month.

Of course, as with all aspects of your sobriety journey, you have to do what feels right for you. I know a lot of people who chose to share what they're doing a bit further down the line or when they hit a significant milestone such as Week 1, Month 1 or Day 50, and I also know others who, like me, used their social media posts for ongoing daily accountability.

As in many areas of life, making yourself accountable has been shown to reap rewards. Let's face it – if you tell absolutely no one that you are trying not to drink, it's going to be a lot easier to give up when it gets hard. And also, if no one knows what you are trying to achieve, you are not going to have that all-important cheer squad or people to celebrate with and tell you how amazingly well you are doing when you get through a difficult week or hit those milestones.

COMMUNITY

Never underestimate the power of community. Your cheer squad is key but there is a whole sober community out there ready to welcome you and offer you support if that's what you want to do.

When I committed to not drinking a sniff of alcohol for 100 days, I knew I couldn't do it solo, that my willpower might waiver, so I decided to sign up to an online community and threw myself into their 90-day challenge. I'll be forever grateful to Andy Ramage and Ruari Fairbairns for One Year No Beer – because if I hadn't signed up to their challenge (while pissed!) one Saturday night, there's not a cat in hell's chance I'd be sharing this with you now and I'm so very grateful I joined when I did.

There are many online and in-person communities you can join and it's so important to find what works for you. We've had guests on the podcast sharing their stories of success with Alcoholics Anonymous (AA); other people I know have joined women-only platforms and some have found their tribe in a Facebook group that might be connected to one of the quit-lit books listed on page 245. Find what works for you, stick with the connections that feel good and lose the ones that don't.

But keep an open mind and do try it out. Finding a gang of people who are going through the same things as you and can

"Never underestimate the power of community"

cheer you on is so, so valuable, particularly, but not exclusively, if you ever feel like you are the only you know who isn't drinking or is trying to address your issues around drinking. And let's face it: if you want to change your relationship with alcohol and ultimately stop drinking, you're not going to get the results you're striving for if you just keep doing what you've always done – and this includes going it alone. Joining a community of like-minded individuals is often the missing piece of the AF jigsaw so if it's something you've resisted previously now is the time to do things differently. It may just be the key to AF success!

You can trust me when I say this as I was someone who had zero understanding about the power of connection at the start of my own booze-free journey. In fact, I would go so far as to say that I actually didn't *want* to connect with anyone. Truthfully, I didn't really know *how* to connect as all my previous socialising had been with people familiar to me with alcohol at the centre of it all. How on earth do you chat to not just NEW people but new SOBER people? It sounded like the stuff of sober nightmares and no way on earth was this going to be for me. I didn't know where to start. But even so ... I threw myself in and I just started.

Three weeks into not drinking and still feeling hugely uncomfortable with every single aspect of it all, I plucked up the courage to attend a one-day conference in Manchester, all to do with not drinking. It was hosted by the online group I'd joined and my decision to go (even though I was DREADING it) was all part of my plan to throw myself in to everything and anything connected with alcohol-free life. You so often hear motivational speakers talk about comfort zones and how you need to step out of them, break them, smash them … well for me, this was one of the most uncomfortable things I did in early sobriety but it also turned out to be one of the best.

I genuinely felt sick at the prospect of it. Would it be weird? Who even goes to stuff like this? How do I cope with the nerves? What if people think I'm bonkers?! Why am I even doing this? But I was twenty-one days in and I had nothing to lose, apart from the cost of my ticket if it turned out to be abysmal.

It didn't. It turned out to be a day of glorious connection, of meeting other people who were wanting to remove the booze and of hearing from others who were much further on and were loving living a sober life. I was fascinated by their stories and curious to understand how they navigated a world where you're usually the odd one out if you're not drinking. By the end of the event, I was genuinely excited, feeling positive and proud that I'd plucked up the courage to go along. I made some wonderful new connections, some of whom are still with me to this day.

It IS nerve-racking meeting new people and trying new things but it's all part of the process. Finding a community of people who absolutely get it, to whom you don't have to explain that you're 'not drinking for a while' or 'trying being sober', is a magical and hugely helpful thing. I firmly believe that once you connect with others just like you, that's where you grow. The growth can be personal and/or professional and is connected to confidence, but once you bite the bullet and do

" Once you connect with others just like you, that's where you grow " things you've never done before the only regret you'll have is not doing it sooner!

You do not need to be addicted to alcohol, or *anything* for that matter, to benefit from human connection. Connection is key. And connection is everything. You do not have to do this on your own. It's true that the road to an alcohol-free life can be a lonely one at times and that's why it's vital to make new connections with people doing what you're doing. For so many, connection is the missing link. It's that final piece of the alcohol-free jigsaw and once it clicks it can mean the difference between being stuck in the cycle of drinking or reaching a place where you know you're totally done.

When you find your tribe and connect with those who get it, that will keep you buoyed when things are tough, or help you share the joy and achievement when you hit those milestones. It's important to surround yourself with a supportive community as that will make your sobriety go the distance.

You're not the only person who drinks and you're not the only person reading this book. If you're feeling a bit worried, nervous, lonely and isolated, you don't need to be. If the thought of joining a community feels a little overwhelming at this stage just hold that thought for now as there are other ways to hear from people on the same journey as you online, without you having to interact yourself just yet.

SOCIAL MEDIA

If you're on social media there are so many ways that you can use it to help you in your AF journey.

Firstly, and most simply, making a few tweaks and changes to your social media feeds can help massively with your mindset when it comes to not drinking. I began by removing all the 'mummy drinking culture' and 'why women drink' accounts and swapped them for inspiring sober socials instead.

I didn't even know how much of a sober community existed on social media until I stopped drinking and began to actively look for AF content. I couldn't believe what was out there. I discovered so many inspiring, friendly and relatable accounts from content creators who'd already walked the path and were now on the other side and loving AF life. That proved to be another useful tool for helping to keep me on track, as it gave me something to read or watch if I was feeling a bit wobbly or as if I was the only person in the world who wasn't drinking.

The algorithms responded and soon my feed began to be flooded with stuff that made sense for what I was trying to achieve. My social media feed began to throw AF and sober content my way. Adverts for online communities. Alcohol-free drinks. Stories from people who were now living happy and fulfilled lives after removing the booze. Book recommendations. A range of positive content continued appearing in my feeds, and eventually these strange little sober seeds that had been planted

"When you find your tribe and connect with those who get it, that will keep you buoyed when things are tough" began to flourish and grow and ultimately led me to where I am today.

Discovering sober socials was a huge benefit for me at the start and even to this day, several years, later I'm still very much connected to some of the original accounts I started to follow. For me, it's all about the accounts that make me laugh and that normalise sobriety. Find what you like and if you feel comfortable commenting and interacting, I would recommend that you do so. You never know, you might make a few AF friends in the process, as social media is another really useful way to connect with others. At the very least, the algorithms will start to send more AF content your way and before you know it, you will know about a load of like-minded individuals who are following the same path as you. Some of the best connections I've made in sobriety have been online!

I had been hugely vocal about my drinking on social media ('It's always gin o'clock somewhere!' *cringe*), but this time I decided to use it to become very vocal about my NOT drinking too. I began to share what I was doing and how it was making me feel across my personal social media as a way of holding myself accountable. I soon found that sharing my little wins and regular rubbish days was helping others who were in the same boat, and in turn their interactions supported me; this process of connection was what somehow led to the creation of our own online Over the Influence (OTI) support community. Going back to the idea of accountability, once you've put it out there, you're instantly accountable and you're much less likely to pick up a drink.

It's about finding out what works for you, what you're comfortable sharing online and how much time you're happy to spend scrolling and using social media.

I know a lot of people who've started their own sober social media accounts both for accountability and to motivate others. Some of these people have put themselves out there from Day 1, complete with name and profile picture, while others have wanted to remain anonymous.

I joined an online community for moral support before one of my thirty-day challenges, but I didn't fully engage. I suppose you could say I was a little bit half-arsed about the whole thing. But still, I recognised that there was something magical about this group. I returned to this very same online community a couple of months later for the start of my 'attempt proper' and this is where everything began to change, one post, one like, one comment and one connection at a time. That's also how I ended up at the sober conference in Manchester, completely out of my comfort zone.

As I keep saying (because it's true!), you need to set aside any pre-conceptions you may have, park your reservations, give yourself a chance and, yet again, ask yourself what's the worst that could happen?

QUIT-LIT

If you are enjoying this book and would like to read more about life alcohol-free or even the more sciency side of what alcohol does to our bodies and brains, or how addiction works, then you are going to be very pleased to hear that there's a lot more out there that you can immerse yourself in. In fact, this type of material has a name: quit-lit. Quit-lit is the broad title given to books, like this, which are all about quitting drinking. There is SO much amazing writing available. As with the socials, I didn't even know it was a 'thing' until I stopped drinking and decided to throw myself head over (usually lost) heels into trying life without it.

Turn to page 245 for some suggestions.

If you're interested, the first quit-lit book I ever read was Catherine Gray's *The Unexpected Joy of Being Sober*. It hit me like a freight train. I saw so much of myself in what Catherine shared and I felt massively connected to her story. It was honest, inspiring, friendly and funny and it gave me so much hope that there was life on the other side of drinking.

PODCASTS

Podcasts are an amazing and free resource for connection and inspiration. There's nothing quite like hearing a situation very similar to yours being described by other people on a public platform. There's so much power and opportunity here – shared stories create bonds, a feeling of recognition and can really help you to keep going. The person you are listening to might be in a different part of the world to you but there's comfort to be found in knowing that they have been where you are and, more importantly, they're now on their other side of it and giving you inspiration, motivation and hope.

There's an amazing stack of superb sober content to listen to, so wherever you download your audio from, fill your ears with as much as possible and find the type of content and style of podcast that you find relatable, enjoyable and fun.

Of course, I'd highly recommend plugging yourself into one of our very own Over the Influence podcast episodes for an hour to hear an inspiring story from someone who might be just like you. Ben and I adore wanging on about AF life week in week out and we're incredibly passionate about what we do. We very much focus on the future and the positives rather than harking back to the past and the associated negatives. We're very northern and we laugh a lot. We would love you to connect with us and our guests! And who knows – you might be one of our special guests a bit further down the line if you fancy joining us to shout about the many benefits of an AF life!

• • •

So think about how you can add the tools I have described in this section into your own personalised AF toolkit. Find a community, think about what forms of accountability could work in your life and how you can use these to motivate you. Have a browse through social media and download some podcasts ready for your commute or morning walk. Check out the reading list on page 245 if reading is what's working for you.

"Give yourself a chance and ask yourself, what's the worst that could happen?"

I understand if you want to keep your drinking as your business but as with everything it's completely up to you. It's 100 per cent your choice. I would just urge you not to dismiss anything out of hand as 'not for me' at this stage in your journey until you've given it some serious thought. Confiding in a trusted friend or a family member, connecting with an alcohol-free support group (never worry this makes it look like you're telling the world you've got a problem!) or interacting with sober accounts on social media can help massively. You will feel less alone and more positively connected with others who understand.

What it all comes down to is remembering that human connection is powerful in all areas of life. In sobriety it is everything. Without it, you can find yourself floundering by yourself wondering why on earth you're bothering. With it you can unlock a whole new world that exists on the other side of alcohol.

CHAPTER 13

The fifty-day questionnaire

At the beginning of the book, I asked you to think about and note down how you were feeling about the part booze was playing in your life and to list some of the areas you hoped would improve when you removed it.

Well, CONGRATULATIONS!! You are halfway through your magical 100 days booze-free. The first, most important thing to do is to give yourself a huge pat on the back. This is an incredible achievement and you deserve to feel so proud of yourself. There are so many people who are thinking about doing this and haven't quite found the courage to try it. But you are living it. WELL DONE! What treat do you have planned to celebrate this momentous milestone?

Now I want you to take some time to reflect, to think about where improvements are being made and the positive changes in your life you're starting to enjoy. Make sure you note down your feelings as well.

The questions on page 161 are intended as prompts to help you do this, but however you want to approach this is fine. I would just urge you to take the step of writing it down – on paper, or on your computer, tablet or phone. Seeing it set out like this can make all the difference.

Compare how you feel now to how to felt when you started out:

- What's going well for you?

- What small improvements are you noticing in day-to-day life?

- What areas are you struggling with?

- Think about a time when you found it really hard and yet you managed to carry on. What helped most in these moments or days?

- How successfully have you been able to anticipate your triggers? Have these changed at all?

- Think about a time when you were dreading something, or anticipating a big challenge to your sobriety, and it was actually much easier than you expected. What happened and helped?

- Is there anything that has helped you that you never would have guessed before you started?

ALLISON'S STORY

After graduating high school, I discovered how much fun alcohol could be. In my early twenties, I was a typical party girl, supporting myself with a full-time job. At twenty-five, I became pregnant with my daughter and knew I had to stop partying to be a mom, which I did effortlessly.

In 2009, I found myself unhappy in my marriage and reconnected with old party friends through Facebook. This rekindled my enjoyment of drinking and socialising. Eventually, I split with my husband and began a relationship with one of these friends. My drinking quickly escalated and as my tolerance grew, so did my daily alcohol intake. I found myself adding shots when beer wasn't enough.

I realised I needed to cut back but I found it very difficult to moderate my drinking. I set rules for myself about which nights I was allowed to drink, tried switching to wine and attempted to limit the number of drinks. None of these strategies worked. I woke up hating myself and I swore off alcohol every morning, but by 2 p.m., I would find a reason to drink. I was miserable. This cycle continued for eight years until I left the relationship I was in.

In my quest to quit or reduce drinking, I read books on quitting alcohol, recovery memoirs and joined an online support group.

A few years later, despite cutting back, alcohol still dominated my thoughts, and even one night of drinking left me wrecked for days.

I had a light bulb moment when I heard sobriety described not as a punishment but as a glorious gift. I stopped drinking immediately and I haven't looked back. Sobriety has indeed been glorious; the best thing I have done for myself.

My relationships with family have improved, I've taken up sewing voraciously and I started attending AA meetings to work through the 12 steps and experience fellowship in my community. I'm excited to see where that takes me.

I know I'll never drink alcohol again. It's actually a relief knowing I'll never have to worry about whether or not I should drink for any reason – that alone was exhausting. Plus, my grandkids will never know me as a drinker which is precious to me.

CHAPTER 14

What longer-term advantages can I look forward to?

YOUR HEALTH

I promised at the start of the book that at no point was I going to hector you or to try to make you feel bad about drinking. And I really don't want to go on about the health implications of drinking alcohol, but now you are making such great progress I think it's well worth taking a minute to reflect on the big favour you are doing for your body and your future health.

The unavoidable fact is that drinking alcohol causes cancer. The detrimental effects make for incredibly (excuse the pun) sobering reading.

- When we drink alcohol, our bodies turn it into a chemical, called acetaldehyde. Acetaldehyde can damage our cells and can also stop cells from repairing this damage.
- Alcohol can increase the levels of some hormones in our bodies such as oestrogen and insulin. Hormones are chemical messengers, and higher levels of oestrogen and insulin can make cells divide more often. This increases the chance that cancer will develop.

- Alcohol can make it easier for cells in the mouth and throat to absorb harmful chemicals that cause damage.

Remember, it's the alcohol itself that damages your body, even small amounts. It doesn't matter whether you drink beer, wine or spirits. All types of alcohol can cause cancer. There are plenty of tricks that people claim 'cure' hangovers. But even if they work for your hangover, they don't reverse the damage caused from drinking alcohol.

According to Cancer Research UK, drinking alcohol causes seven types of cancer. These include:

- Breast cancer and bowel cancer (two of the most common types)
- Mouth cancer
- Some types of throat cancer: oesophagus (food pipe), larynx (voice box) and pharynx (upper throat)
- Liver cancer

GOOD SLEEP

Of course, getting a good night's sleep is a major pillar of health and wellbeing. There is nothing quite like sober sleep and these days nothing gives me greater joy than an early night followed by a fresh early morning! And if you are a night owl who has no intention of going to bed before midnight, it's still so much easier and you will feel so much better not to have to peel yourself off the mattress the next morning because you've had a fitful, booze-addled night's sleep. I dread to think how many precious sleep hours I've thrown away thanks to booze and if this is you too, rest assured you will eventually get them back.

You might at first experience some weird drinking dreams. I can offer no credible or scientific explanation for this. All I know is that I woke up panicked before the absolute relief of knowing I had in fact gone to bed sober kicked in! Remember, you can't undo months or years of boozing overnight. It takes time and patience.

A good night's sleep = a fabulously fresh morning and I can 100 per cent guarantee that you will NEVER tire of the feeling! Channel that inner smug to the max and you'll soon have others asking you why you're smiling inanely, how come you're so fresh faced and urging you to share your secrets!

DIET AND EXERCISE

You may lose some weight of course, particularly considering the calories you're not going to be pouring down your neck. However, as a fifty-year-old chonky menopausal woman sporting a thick middle section that will not deflate or change shape no matter how hard I try, I'm in no position at all to be dishing out health and fitness advice or motivational gubbins.

What I can share with you is that, despite weighing more now than I did as a drinker, I'm the happiest I've ever been with the way I look and feel. I am fitter, more active and I have a

"Remember, slow and steady wins the race!"

much better relationship with food. I look back on photos from my drinking days and compare them to now and even though there's been no weight loss, I've deflated and lost the boozy bloat.

Drinking used to totally screw with my eating habits and I'd often skip meals or eat less so I could drink more. I'd never have a dessert if I was eating out at a restaurant with the family and would instead use that time to have more wine while they tucked into their puddings. Eating out was less about the food and more about how much I could drink. I was sick so often through drinking that it's no wonder I weighed considerably less than I do now. To me, eating was cheating and it was a crime to waste valuable calories on food when you could save them to drink instead. I now cringe to think of what I was putting my body through.

I know loads of people who've made exercise part of their alcohol-free (AF) routine and consequently lost weight. There are so many other ways you can measure your AF success, however, than by the numbers on the scales, and others will soon be asking future you what the secret is to your newly found glow!

Don't put too much pressure on yourself to become a healthy-eating, new-language-learning, 10k-running, gym-loving, sunrise-chasing, sober superstar all at once. If all you do during your first 100 days is simply not drink and eat considerably more cake and sweets than you've ever done before, give yourself the biggest pat on the back and have another slice because you're already winning. Carry on past 100 days, feel the benefits accumulating and then it will become so easy to make positive choices about what you eat and how often you exercise. It's so much easier to get out of the door for that walk/run/yoga session when you are already feeling positive and upbeat. It doesn't all have to happen at once. Remember, slow and steady wins the race!

I'm definitely more tortoise than hare, which was glaringly evident in my sub-seven-hour London Marathon in 2022. By sub, I mean 6:59:59! I still eat too much cake and too many sweets, I'll never ditch the caffeine, I enjoy hiking and being outdoors by the coast and I exercise at the gym occasionally when I decide I'm in the mood. There's no right or wrong way to do any of this. All you need to do is what feels right for you.

A BETTER PERIMENOPAUSE

If you're reading this as a woman in mid-life who's been drinking regularly for a good number of years and you're now in the madly confusing throes of perimenopause, it's great to have you here! Welcome to a Very Rubbish Club! I see you, I hear you and I feel your befuddled pain! If you are a woman who is not at that stage yet, you might want to stay with me here anyway as it's still good to hear this subject talked about. If you are a man then this is what some of the ladies in your life might be going through, so I urge you to do the gentlemanly thing and listen up for a moment rather than skipping onto the next section. If you are a lady who has made it through to the other side then I salute you.

There's something in the region of ninety – yes NINETY – symptoms of perimenopause and menopause. Is it any wonder

"There's no right or wrong way to do any of this. All you need to do is what feels right for you" that we women can feel like we're losing the actual plot when we hit our mid forties?! Especially if we're using booze to medicate and mask a whole load of stuff we've not encountered before. All of a sudden, we can find ourselves dealing with crushing anxiety for possibly the first time in our lives and we haven't got a clue why. Family may find themselves taking the brunt of brutal mood swings because of our hormone changes; issues with concentration and memory loss – a.k.a. the hell that is brain fog – can impede working life and what were previously simple day-to-day tasks. New aches and pains from top to toe mysteriously appear from nowhere despite us not having started a new exercise regime; we often have difficulty sleeping and night sweats might wake us up when we finally drop off. Oh, and there may be hot flushes just when we least expect them, or frequent headaches or migraines knocking us for six. There's that bloody awful weight gain around the middle that seemingly appears overnight and just will not budge no matter how hard we try to shift it and the changes in our skin ... dry skin, saggy skin, hairy skin, blotchy skin. Urgh. Urinary infections are painful, bladder issues are embarrassing, hair can fall out in clumps from our heads and yet we also find ourselves using our mobile phone torchlights in the mirror to chase the new stubby chin and cheek hairs with tweezers that are popping up at an alarming rate! We have sore gums, dry eyeballs and heart palpitations and that, my friend, is just for starters! I'm exhausted just writing that! (Did I mention that you can feel exhausted all the time too?)

You don't need to be Einstein to figure out that if you have added into this mix a daily wine habit or regular weekend binge drinking then you can very easily create the perfect mental and physical health shit storm for yourself where you literally will not know your arse from your elbow. So many of the unpleasant effects alcohol causes are mirrored and made worse during perimenopause. So hands down the best chance you can give yourself to work through all above the above and then some is to take alcohol out of the equation.

Remove the booze, look at the symptoms you're left with and you'll then know exactly what you're dealing with going forward. You can then seek any medical help you need, clear in the distinction between what's the fault of your hormones and what was caused by booze. It's truly the best gift of self-care you can give to yourself.

You don't need to feel shit through your forties and continue in the same vein into your fifties. Give yourself a break. There's so much more to midlife than being stuck on the relentless hangover hamster wheel of hell wondering why you're feeling crap most days. Removing the booze will not only give you the mental lift that you need, it will also help you navigate what might be years of perimenopause with clarity. You absolutely deserve to feel good about yourself and stopping drinking will allow that to happen slowly but surely.

YOUR EMOTIONAL WELLBEING

Breaking News Shocker! I'm not a medical professional or psychologist – I'm simply a retired professional ex-drinker who's been there, done that and spilled wine down the T-shirt more times than I care to remember. But I can tell you for sure that – in the long run, if not on Day 1, or even Week 2 – not drinking is so good for your mood and your overall wellbeing.

- Firstly, there's the pride you feel in choosing to put yourself before booze day after day after day. This will make your heart swell.
- Then there are the lots of little positive nods of recognition from those who love you dearly and who will notice the change in you as your confidence grows and you have so much more energy to focus on the things that are important to you.
- Yes, there can be moments when you've no idea why you're crying again and others when you're blubbing happy tears of relief that you're no longer drinking or just because you're crying laughing with friends and family you hold close to your heart. My advice is just to go with it – it's part of the process!
- Once you start to get towards the end of your (first?!) 100 days, you should notice your mood improving and your anxiety levels dropping. And if you don't? Well, we started this journey because we recognised

"Not drinking is so good for your mood and your overall wellbeing" that problems don't go away if you ignore them. This presents an opportunity to seek help for anything that is bothering you, with the renewed strength that comes from having proof in front of your eyes that you can face difficult things and get through them.

In early sobriety, I used to cry while walking by the beach at 5 a.m … tears of relief that I was ACTUALLY DOING THIS REALLY HARD THING. And there's nothing quite like sunrise with one of the kids up a mountain. Nothing. The physical and mental health benefits of removing alcohol are endless and often surprising, and it is so worth working hard to make it feel good.

FRIENDSHIPS

Some friends may think your being sober is a boring lifestyle choice, and that's their prerogative. But as we talked about in the section about community (see page 145 for a reminder), there is always the option of connecting with others in the same boat as yourself for that solidarity and collective moral support. You feel far less alone and there's nothing more motivating than hearing from people who are on a similar journey to you. I have made so many amazing new friends thanks to my decision to break up with booze.

If some of your old friends really don't get it then it might be time to move on because I can guarantee you the new ones you make in sobriety *will* get it. There's no judgement or questioning, just camaraderie and understanding in the sober community! One of our community members, Rich, shared a saying that stuck with me: 'If you want to go fast, go alone. If you want to go far, go together.'

As well as making new connections in the future, you may well find that you have the time and energy to renew old ones too. Think about friends you've lost touch with over the years who you'd like to pick up with again. I spent YEARS saying to one old school friend 'Oh, we must get together …', 'Let's go for a drink …', 'Catch up at Christmas … ?'. How many times do you do that before you realise the best part of five years has passed? But somehow, I never made the effort. To be honest, more often than not it meant we'd have to drive to meet somewhere in the middle and no way was I going to forfeit my wine for anyone! I used to put alcohol before so many other things, things that were much more important than a large glass or two of pinot. But when I stopped drinking – guess what? I did make the effort and it's been ace reconnecting again and we now catch up as often as we can.

You will learn which friendships were built on a foundation of alcohol and you will discover who loves you for exactly who you are. You will also be so much better at showing up for your friends when your social interactions don't revolve around alcohol. Oversharing after a few glasses is not the same as building lasting, honest relationships based on trust and genuine care for someone.

There are no hard and fast rules to follow and your experiences of how friendship changes may look very different to those of the next person. Though, having said that, it's a bit of a cliché but it's so true: you really do find out who your true friends are when you decide to stop drinking and live life differently. Hold on dearly to the ones who are cheerleading your progress and allow the ones who aren't to move on.

A POSITIVE IMPACT ON OTHERS

The clarity of sobriety shone the brightest light on what a 'pusher' I was when it came to drinking. I always drank way too fast and would often be opening another bottle while family members would happily still be on their first glass. Even though it was glaringly obvious I drank like a fish, in my head I didn't want to stand out so would always be offering more drinks and topping up other people's glasses. It's been so interesting to observe how others in my family drink now when we get together for the annual Boxing Day buffet or the big summer BBQ – in a nutshell, they hardly touch it. No one's arsed. If my mum wants a G&T she'll have one and that'll be her done for the next three months. If either of my brothers fancy a beer, they'll have one. Maybe a couple. What they no longer have to deal with is their drunk older sister pushing them to neck more, keep up and then start on the shots and shorts!

My eldest kids, both in their twenties, rarely drink these days. Again, they're just not particularly interested in alcohol, which is a really wonderful position to be in! I've no doubt that my decision to stop drinking has also had a hugely positive impact on them too. I'm not a finger-wagging sober parent that believes they shouldn't drink – it's absolutely their choice – but what they have seen over the years is how my life, and theirs, has changed for the better because booze no longer features, and I've also been able to show them you don't need it to have fun and enjoy life!

Even if you don't have kids, when others around you see how you have taken the bull by the horns and sorted out an issue that was bothering you, that's going to have an impact. So many people have confessed to me their concerns around their drinking. That they feel comfortable to do so, and the fact that I am now in a position where I may be able to offer helpful advice (rather than topping up their glass), absolutely warms my cockles.

REDISCOVERING TALENTS AND PASSIONS

When I was a drinker, I used to wholeheartedly take the piss out of anything not connected to alcohol. Afternoon TEA? Why would you unless Prosecco was included? Amateur dramatics? How dull. Early morning beach walks? I'd rather be in bed. Sunrise up a mountain? See above. The thing with sobriety is you will find yourself making changes (lots of them exciting ones!) in order for this to work and for it to begin to feel good for you. Remember: you are not just removing booze, you are creating a space you can fill with whatever you want to be in your life instead.

Clare Pooley, author of the amazing *The Sober Diaries*, joined us on the podcast to share her own incredible and

"You are not just removing booze, you are creating a space to fill with all the things you want to be in your life instead" inspiring sobriety journey. One thing that really resonated with me was her observation that sobriety uncovers who you really are and also in many ways takes you right back to who you were as a child. Clare loved writing when she was younger. She removed booze as an adult and rediscovered her amazing ability that had been lying dormant for years.

Another guest we spoke to, a fantastic guy called Paul Lock, found out that he was a world-class artist once he stopped drinking. Allie, a community member in the States who shared her alcohol-free journey in the previous chapter, put down the glass and picked up her quilting tools. She's loving her long-lost hobby once again.

NEW HOBBIES AND EXPERIENCES

We've talked about time, about how drinking alcohol can steal so much of it, whether you are drinking, thinking about drinking, or recovering from drinking. Now you can have all of that time back! You can replace your evening tipple time with a new activity or hobby. You can extend the free time across your weekend by choosing not to drink on a Friday and Saturday night – you'll get your mornings back! It's that simple.

Throw yourself in to something completely bonkers or, if you'd rather play it safe at first, test the waters with a new hobby or pick up an old one that might have previously got in the way of your drinking. Just give it a go because you can't get any of this wrong.

Back in 2022, when I'd have been around three and a half years sober, BBC Radio Lancashire sent me along to record a piece at the auditions for *Calendar Girls the Musical* which was being staged by the Preston Musical Comedy Society! If you've seen the original *Calendar Girls* film starring Helen Mirren and Julie Walters from 2003, you'll know the incredible story of a group of women from Yorkshire who stripped off for a charity calendar. As part of the piece I was recording for my radio show, I 'auditioned' for the role of Marie, the bossy chairwoman of the Women's Institute. I inadvertently and sort of accidentally nailed the audition and somehow got the part!

The four months that followed were genuinely some of the best I've ever had. It was immense fun and I was made to feel so warmly welcome as a brand new member of the group despite having so much to learn. Everything was new, overwhelming and nerve-wracking. But I learned my lines, I sang my heart out and I loved making new friends with the rest of the cast and crew. I was SO far out of my comfort zone it was painful but it was truly one of the best experiences of my life and one I'm so very grateful for. I will never forget walking out on the stage and seeing my entire family laughing and clapping on the front row.

I STILL can't believe I did it. But that's another bit of the magic of quitting drinking … it makes you brave!

"Another bit of the magic of quitting drinking is it makes you brave!"

JUST NOT DRINKING FEELS GOOD!

Do you remember the wonderful film *The Wizard of Oz* starring Judy Garland? To this day, it's still one of my all-time favourites. I can remember watching it for the first time as a child in the late 1970s and the way it made me feel. I was mesmerised by Dorothy and her cute little dog, Toto, and I fell in love with Scarecrow, The Tin Man, The Cowardly Lion and the Munchkins. The film starts off in black and white before exploding into glorious technicolor when Dorothy's house lands in Oz and she says 'Toto, I've a feeling we're not in Kansas anymore …'. THAT scene, that change, that transition to bright colour from black and white is exactly what sobriety looked like for me in a nutshell. That's how I eventually felt when the exhaustion and frustration finally lifted … like Dorothy stepping into Oz. The raging storm had passed and it had been replaced by an unusual and unfamiliar calm. It was starting to feel good and I could sense adventure ahead. All I had to do was to keep choosing not to drink and not have that first one. Had I accepted that first drink when offered or chosen to pour myself that first one at home any decision regarding further drinks would've been taken firmly out of my hands.

JONNY'S STORY

My weekend drinking was fun in my teens and twenties. In my thirties, it was at social events with other parents. In my forties, I was regularly drinking at home, and going into my fiftieth year, I was drinking all day every day and sneaking around doing it. It had taken over. I had no energy. I was being sick every morning. I was an empty vessel with no soul. I had nothing to give the people I wanted to give everything to. That's when I knew I had to stop.

I could see what rock bottom looked like, and I was fast approaching it. I stumbled across some alcohol-free (AF) literature, which in turn led me to listening to Sharon hosting the Over the Influence podcast more than two years ago now. I remember exactly where I was and how desperate I felt when that first podcast went on.

I've never looked back. Was it a lifesaver? I don't know and I'm glad I will never find out but what I will say is just knowing I wasn't alone, that I wasn't a failure and there was nothing wrong with me – this is what happens when humans put poison in their body for decades – made all the difference.

I am healthier than I've ever been, and not just physically. Mentally I'm so strong; stronger than I could ever have imagined and I can carry people

...hey need me. I've stepped up when I was ...ded by my family. I'm resilient, funny, caring and smart; all the things I wanted to be. I just needed to remove alcohol. I've repaired relationships with people I hold dear to me and I'm in an infinitely better place. My smiles are real.

More than two years alcohol-free, I can look forward to years of happy booze-free memories, especially as I'm now a grandad. I'm going to take a real shot at this next stage of my life and being AF has a huge part to play in that. Camper van purchased, trips being planned, maybe an early retirement and a decent pension to blow on doing things – real things – not just spending time in a pub dulling my senses and my personality.

CHAPTER 15

What about dating as a sober person?

As my sober journey began long after I got married, I never had to navigate this particular area having recently ditched the booze, but if you are single it may well be something you are thinking about. So I reached out to the Over the Influence community to get their thoughts.

Looking at it logically, *of course* meeting and getting to know someone without alcohol in the mix is a great idea – no more beer googles, no questionable decisions, no hazy memories wondering if you made a tit of yourself in front of someone you fancy. But here we again run into the issue of how ingrained alcohol is in our culture and the fear of other people judging us for not drinking – whether we're worrying they will think we are boring or that they might assume we had some terrible problem and were forced to give up because of it. But this is also where we have to keep a central fact front and centre in our minds: this is about YOU. It's not about anyone else or about pleasing anyone else – it's 100 per cent about you, the way alcohol makes you feel and only your reasons as to why you want to make a change. Your life and how you want it to look is so much more important than the anticipated views (that they may well not hold anyway) of someone you might want to date.

That said, I totally understand if you are looking to date at the moment and you have no idea how you are going to do it without a bit of courage-in-a-glass to get the conversation going, or what you are going to say to someone who asks you out 'for a drink'.

So let's turn to Andy, Cath, Frederica, Holly and Catherine to get the benefit of their experiences.

ANDY – I started dating someone recently and on our first date I drove to Liverpool to meet her. I had one of the best first dates because I was sober. We played crazy golf and then on to loads of really cool bars near the docks – we had a ball! I was more present, had loads of fun and was up dancing, all on the 0% beers.

I had been a little anxious about it but she was so great, asking me if I minded if she was having a drink, which I have no problem with. We have had a further six dates as I write and she is really understanding about me not wanting a drink, which was a concern of mine before we met, as you never know if you're going to be judged once you throw it out there. It's such a relief that it's not a problem.

CATH – I'm OK when I'm out but my big thing was the pre-date, drinking that bottle of wine getting ready and although I'm sure a lot will agree it's the same going to a party, girls' night out or similar, the predrinking calmed me (or so I thought) before that initial meeting.

FREDERICA – Drinking me wasn't really the authentic me. I was out of control in a lot of ways, had very low self-esteem and had gotten myself trapped on the hamster wheel of dating men who were in-your-face pub goers who loved a drink and I thought that's what I liked. After getting sober I realised this really wasn't who I was at all and the men I thought I liked, I really didn't. Sobriety gave me clarity to truly understand who I was and what made me happy and in turn what characteristics I was looking for in a life partner. And I quickly realised booze was not a part of that!

Sobriety gave me the time and space and clarity of mind to work on myself, understand the behaviours that had led me to where I was and work on freeing myself and undoing a lot of ingrained behaviours.

When I did decide to date again, I used the apps but I wasn't fussy at all. Not because I didn't have clear boundaries but because I realised that I hadn't made good choices before so I should let go of any pre-judgements. I think I swiped right on everybody, whether they were fat, thin, tall, short, etc. because I now wanted to get to know people based on their values and characteristics not on their hairline!

I also decided not to do the dinner/drinks thing to begin with. I found the pressure of that quite overwhelming, so I planned dog walks/tea meet ups. A few people were put off by that which was absolutely fine as it showed me that they weren't right for me. I liked the idea of taking the pressure off and just seeing whether there was any chemistry at all before booking in another date that was more 'traditional'.

A big lesson for me is that we spend so much time worrying if people like us but sometimes don't stop to question how much we really like them. When I was drinking, I had no idea whether I liked them or if it was the alcohol. Similarly, I did things and would wonder *Did I do that because I like them or because of the alcohol?* Sobriety is amazing because you know everything you feel is because of you. That red flag is much clearer when you're sober, as are the green flags, and you can hand on heart say that you are making decisions based on your own desires, which is a huge win!

To be honest, I didn't date much because I met my partner very quickly. Obviously it does help that he is also sober, it has been amazing to share this journey with him, but I believe being honest and proud about your sobriety upfront is key! People that are the right people for you will not mind at all and being honest sorts the wheat from the chaff!

HOLLY – I'm in the process of developing a dating app for people who want to go on a sober date! It is not just for people who are sober, but it is for people who are sick of feeling like they have to drink when they go on that first date. I have so many friends who are single and still drink but are no longer using dating apps because they are sick of having to conform to this idea that dates involve alcohol. For some people, it's simply because weekends are precious so they want to go out midweek and they don't want to drink on a work night. I have other friends who are sick of going on dates and the guys rocking up half cut. I'm sure the same goes for men too because a lot of girls drink half a bottle of wine for Dutch courage for a first date. My best friend is single and she said that she would never suggest going for a walk as a first date because it would imply that she is boring. We definitely need to change this idea – there are so many thousands of people who don't want to drink on a date for so many reasons!

CATHERINE – I recently got up the confidence to have a go at sober dating. I've been divorced for over twenty years and in the past, I have hated online dating. I don't think I'd ever been on a date that didn't involve alcohol.

There's the question of 'Is it too soon?', of judging when you are ready. It is often said 'do nothing big in your first year' – in AA, for example, they say you shouldn't date in the first year. Though this will be different for different people. I am 200 days sober and I have just started dating, but I did wonder if I should wait for a year?

If I like the look of somebody (and their profile) I will take a risk of swiping right if they are a drinker. If I am on the fence about somebody and their profile then the 'drinker' sways me to the left. So this says to me that I am OK if the person drinks – if their profile is up to snuff.

The first guy I met up with did drink, was very polite and asked if I minded him drinking. I said no and he said he doesn't drink much anyway.

The second date I went on was for a coffee and river walk. The guy didn't ask why I don't drink and it didn't feel like it is an issue.

I think a lot of single people who have recently given up drinking wonder about sober sex. When you're used to the 'first time' always having had some element of alcohol relaxant involved, you may well be anxious about what might it be like to have sober sex with somebody the first time you jump their bones! I think that's only natural.

* * *

One of the main things I have learned about giving up drinking is how many magical things come your way when you are not operating in a fog of booze or relying on it to grease the wheels of social interaction. It opens the door to knowing who you really are and what you actually want. Realising that you have the strength and confidence to remove alcohol from your life and turn down all offers of a drink is a powerful thing. Yes, on this journey you will have to relearn an awful lot and face some uncomfortable feelings, but what's on the other side makes it so worth it. All of this applies to dating and falling in love too. Let the next person you like see the real you, full of the joys of realising how strong you are for quitting something that was only ever holding you back.

CHAPTER 16

. . . .

How do I get through difficult life stuff without booze?

Have you ever drunk alcohol for a bit of Dutch courage? Had a quick one to take the edge off ahead of a night out or necked a couple of shots to make you feel a tad more confident ahead of meeting new people for the first time? Fake News Alert! There is NOTHING, and I mean nothing, that hands down gives you real courage more than doing anything sober where previously you would have drunk.

But having said that, if you are someone who has used alcohol as a coping mechanism for a long time, even when you feel like you are through the hard part and enjoying a hangover-free existence, life might still suddenly throw you a curveball that makes you feel like you want to drink to deal with it. Because triggers aren't just beer gardens on sunny days or a tray of champagne at a wedding – shit hitting the Dyson Cool Tower can give you the urge to fall back on old, unhelpful habits too.

Nine months into sobriety, I had to deal with the loss of our family business. This was a real make-or-break situation, in which I truly learned what is was to feel all the feels and learn from scratch how to drag myself from a confidence rock-bottom.

I remember a conversation with a lovely friend in her back garden about 18 months or so after we lost the business and she told me she couldn't believe I was tackling this sober: 'You mean you've not even had a couple to deal with it all?'

And luckily, I was far enough into my alcohol-free (AF) journey at this time that I would say in all honesty that I hadn't. Not one. Did I *think* about drinking at a time when everything was going to shit? Of course. I hadn't at this stage even got a year of sobriety under my belt. But what I had (finally!) learned by then is that alcohol would only provide a short-term reprieve. Nothing good was ever going to come from drinking during this difficult time.

Have you ever seen that meme on social media that declares 'NO GREAT STORY EVER STARTED WITH A SALAD!' Well take it from me, no great *success* story ever started with a drink either.

Think about the tough times in your life and how you've navigated them. Has alcohol helped? It might have temporarily numbed out feelings you didn't want to feel at the time or postponed you having to deal with the hand you've been dealt, but honestly, all it does is provide an instant fix for something that more often than not is not going to go away and will require your focused, sober attention at some point.

I managed to drag myself from this crushing, disappointing low to a place where I've never been happier or more fulfilled at work. Was it easy? Hell, no! Was it terrifying? Hell, yes! Did sobriety make it harder? No. Definitely not. Sobriety gave me

"No great success story ever started with a drink"

needed to get through it. A clear head meant
ons and the knowledge that I had managed not to
r nine whole months meant I believed in my ability to
difficult things.

I completely understand that things falling to shit around you can make you want to jump hard on the fuck-it button like nothing else. But if you find yourself in this situation then, please, in the first instance, reach out and tell someone how you feel. Stop, take a deep breath, go back to your 'why' and remind yourself of how strong you have been to achieve what you have.

There is no shame in wanting to drink. Like we keep saying, alcohol is an addictive substance and drinking is hard-wired into our culture. That's not your fault. But you can choose to say no to it. I know you can.

CHAPTER 17

What about booze-free holidays?

don't know about you but the words 'alcohol-free' and 'holiday' were never part of the same sentence in my vocabulary and prior to stopping drinking I honestly couldn't think of anything worse. I mean, when a bit of sunshine in the back garden at home was a potential trigger for me in the early days, imagine how I felt about my first ever alcohol-free (AF) holiday! Holidays – in my misguided view back then – especially those in guaranteed sunshine or all-inclusive (AI) are designed for drinking from the moment the poolside bar opens until one can drink no more. *That's* why we take two weeks off work and spend all that money, right? Drinking all that booze equalled a *relaxing break*.

This might not be your experience at all of course, especially if you are the sort of person who likes outdoorsy, adventure-type holidays. Or, on the other hand, depending on your age, alcohol might have featured in all of your adult mini-breaks, camping trips, staycations or holidays abroad for many years or even decades. In which case, the prospect of holidaying without drinking probably wasn't on your radar until now. Even the mere thought of dipping your toe into an AF trip might have you crying into your *cerveza sin alcohol*, especially if you've already got something booked in those first 100 days of giving sobriety a go and you're feeling nervous, nay TERRIFIED, about how it might be. Yes, of course there are triggers, reminders and hurdles to navigate – likely many more so than in your day-to-day life – and it may be harder to plan when you are somewhere unfamiliar, but aren't you a bit curious to find out what's on the other side of those never-ending holiday drinks?

ALCOHOL ABROAD

Let's just take a moment to weigh up how previous holidays have looked when you've been drinking against how you've felt upon your return.

- How often on holiday have you overdone it during the day and found yourself lacking in motivation and energy to enjoy the evening ahead?

- Have you ever cancelled or postponed a planned morning excursion or trip out because you felt rough or just tired from a later-than-planned night? ('I'm sure the early morning market won't be that good. Let's just go to the supermarket later.')

- In the past, have you promised yourself that you definitely won't overdo it, only to wake up more mornings than you wanted to groggy and dying of thirst, feeling less-than-enthused about the day ahead in the wonderful location you were so looking forward to visiting? If you've been down the frankly miserable and predictable moderation route more times then you care to remember then you'll no doubt be painfully aware that setting yourself rules when it comes to drinking alcohol invariably ends up with them being broken as soon as you've had those first couple of drinks anyway.

- How many holidays have you returned from feeling like you need another holiday (or detox) to get over it and gone back to work feeling more tired and out of it than you did before you left?

Let's say that, maybe for the first time ever in your adult life or for a good few years at least, you're going to commit to zero booze for the duration of your holiday wherever it may be, no matter who you're with and regardless of what you've got planned.

As with anything you tackle for the first time in sobriety, you're going to need a plan. Yes, another one! Otherwise you leave yourself vulnerable to trips and slips when you least expect it. The first thing you need to do is take a deep breath, suck it up and accept that your first holiday without alcohol is not going to be the same as any that you've experienced previously. Even if you are not a heavy drinker, this will be the case. If you have been a 'Yay! Holiday time! All bets are off and let's start with one in the airport at 8 a.m.!' drinker then this break will feel hugely different to others you have been on from start to finish.

If you are reading this and thinking that sounds awful, and that you are going to have to 'deprive' yourself of something you've always seen as one of the 'best bits' of going away, then hold that thought because once you have got your head round this (and that plan in place of course!) you're going to be surprised by how good it can be.

Does this idea of a booze-free break sound daunting? That makes sense. But only at first; this feeling won't last. You're experiencing a fear of the unknown – of not knowing what it will be like and how you will cope. That's natural but it won't last and there are things you can do to help you feel less daunted. I've got some tips for you below in terms of how to plan ahead for a hugely enjoyable booze-free break. But first, as ever, let's just take a moment to think what opportunities are opened up when you uninvite alcohol on your holiday:

- Any late nights will be because the fun you were having made it worth it, and not because the alcohol made you think it was a good idea to carry on.
- When you are not tired and hungover, the mornings open right up and you can do whatever you want with them. What do you fancy? Getting the beach to yourself before the tourists descend? Your pick of the café tables to drink coffee and watch the town come to life? A hike before it gets too hot?

...be being one of first out on the freshly

...omed piste is what appeals?

The way is opened up to a different holiday experience, now you have more time and the money you would have spent on cocktails. Research what's available near where you're staying and consider trying something new. Take a foodie tour? Have a go on a segway? Try a new activity? That's more interesting and adventurous than spending the afternoon at the hotel bar, right?

- And you'll have more energy for these mini adventures. If you're going with kids, they will love the new, energetic you, who is present, more relaxed and up for fun. If you're not, then *you* will love the new energetic you!

- There's honestly nothing quite like the freedom you feel when you make the choice to turn down each and every drink. (I was asked recently to sum up AF life using only one word and this was the word I chose. FREEDOM.) When you're not drinking on holiday you're not tied. You can do what you want when you want without twitching on your sun lounger towards cocktail o'clock; there's the option to drive and explore new places by car and you don't have to worry about taxis. There is such liberation in rewriting your own story and being free to do whatever you wish.

- And when you get home you will be well-rested (rather than jaded and foggy from too many late nights and shots of local spirits), healthy and glowing. In other words, how we always imagine we will be after that break we are looking forward to, but that strangely never materialises when we have spent two weeks drinking every day …

Never in my life before have I enjoyed holidays with family and friends as much as when doing them sober. My amazing friends Anna, Jeanette and Shani (the BEST AF cheerleading team in all of the land!) took me to Milan as an early birthday surprise for my fiftieth in September 2023. They had a few wines, I didn't, and we all had The Best Time Ever. I spent my actual big birthday in Barbados a month later with my closest family. I've never been as grateful to be sober. It was nothing short of perfect and I loved – and will always remember – every single sober minute with those I care about the most. I spent the New Year in Iceland with my husband, our youngest, my best friend and her family and was completely present for every chaotic, crazy and bitterly cold moment. Alcohol wouldn't have added anything – in fact, still-drinking me would not have been able to appreciate all the special moments nearly so much. It's mad to think that I once believed it was impossible to go on holiday and not have a drink.

Before you go away, go back to that original plan you made and think how you might need to develop it to help you have a successful AF holiday. What could prove to be your triggers? The key is to manage your expectations and be ready for the curveballs.

Here are some tips based on my experiences of my first trips away booze-free:

1. Share what you're doing with those you're going on holiday with before you go. Forewarned is forearmed! It'll save any uncomfortable discussions on arrival and you've confidently set out your stall from the start.

2. If you're flying, find out in advance what the food (or shopping!) options are airside so you have somewhere in mind to wait for your gate and can give the busy airport bar a swerve. What treat are you going to replace that airport beer or glass of fizz with?

3. If your AF options on holiday are limited, ask if the bar person can make you something 'off menu'. You may well find a delicious fruit juice or AF version of the local mulled wine materialises.

4. If the restaurant staff bring complimentary shots or liqueurs with the bill, politely decline or pass it to someone else. You can't avoid alcohol on holiday, especially if you're with others who are drinking, but you can put boundaries in place to keep you on track.

5. If your budget allows it (although think of the money you're saving by not spending it at the bar!), consider booking some early morning trips or excursions. If you've got a reason to get up and out, you're making yourself far more accountable and you'll be much less likely to throw in the (beach) towel. Appoint yourself

Head of Activities and do some stuff you've never done on holiday before!

6. Is there anything from your routine at home that will help you on holiday? For example, a particular herbal tea you enjoy in the evening or a relaxing bath oil?

7. If you're on holiday with a group and you think some of them may kick on to the early hours, make sure you have a brilliant book/great podcast/boxset ready to go, so if you're done with the evening but not ready for bed, you still have something nice to look forward to back at the hotel, villa or apartment.

8. If you are going away with a group, don't assume that everyone else will want to be out all night. When people see that you are confidently heading home when you're done, rather than forcing the fun, and waking up fresh and ready to go the next day, you may well find that others are relieved and happy to follow your example.

Finally, just remember that you are in new territory and embarking on a new adventure … and this is exciting! By repeatedly choosing not to drink you're not going to waste a single minute of your holiday on thinking about drinking, deciding what and how much you're drinking, actually drinking, drinking too much, being ill from drinking then recovering from drinking by drinking. Remind yourself every single day that it's not about giving anything up but about everything you gain. Once alcohol is removed, your holidays become so much more about the people and the places. AF holidays hit different and once you've learned how to navigate them, you'll realise they're actually the stuff of dreams.

You will return home feeling proud, human and fabulous. It's a huge achievement to change the narrative you've previously lived by and it's a really big deal to make that decision to do life differently. Keep this in the back of your mind and always play it forward. Can you really imagine waking up on holiday feeling clear headed and ready to go, but wishing you'd got sloshed the night before?

Motivational quote alert: if you want something you've never had you've got to do something you've never done.

SUSAN'S STORY

I stopped drinking in 2021. I didn't realise at the time that it was going to be for good but deep down I knew that's what I wanted, even though I was reluctant to acknowledge it. I couldn't imagine a life without alcohol.

In my early twenties, I was a weekend binge drinker, but as I headed into my thirties my drinking escalated and I became a daily wine drinker. I worked hard and it was easy to tell myself I deserved a drink after a busy day. This carried on for decades.

I would happily acknowledge that I was a heavy drinker. I made some stupid and unsafe decisions when I was single and there are things I have done when I was pissed that I am ashamed of or regret. There were times when I questioned if I was an 'alcoholic'. But I felt that I held life together sufficiently successfully to believe that alcohol was not causing me a problem big enough that I needed to do something about it.

As I headed into my fifties, I hit the menopause, which impacted my sleep and increased my anxiety significantly. I was a daily bottle-of-wine drinker with more at weekends at that point. From 2019, I stopped drinking every day and became a weekly binge drinker instead. This to me was moderation and success! But I was sick of having so many rules around alcohol and I knew that my drinking levels were still very unhealthy.

After several short stints of not drinking, I finally decided to take an extended break from alcohol. It wasn't easy and I devoured podcasts and quit-lit. Within a week, I was feeling the benefits of reduced head chatter and a clearer mind. My sleep improved as did my anxiety.

I have stopped smoking, taken up wild swimming, run half marathons and hiked up mountains since I stopped drinking. I took early retirement, moved to the coast and retrained as a coach. The future looks gentler and kinder, now I have the clarity of mind to deal with life's issues without using alcohol. I also feel free from the restrictions that alcohol put on me. I also now know I am no longer committing slow suicide, which is how I sometimes felt before.

CHAPTER 18

What do I do if it goes wrong?

"If you trip up and have a drink, the most important thing is not to give up"

The first thing I want to say here is that not succeeding at first isn't failure, it's learning. I really hope you have discovered the unexpected joys (and some expected ones!) and it's all going tickety boo. But let's face it, it's not always that simple. I've shared how many times I did Sober October and thirty-day challenges (with mixed success!) before I got to the point where I gave it my all and gave up for good. *I know* that it's not always easy.

For one, life, and the curveballs it throws, continues regardless and just because you've removed alcohol doesn't mean you've magically smoothed life's often rocky path, with its problems and pitfalls. Of course you haven't. In fact, the chances are you've uncovered stuff you weren't even bargaining for and exposed them to the full sober light of day. You've ripped off the sticking plaster you may have had in place for a while to distract you from things you've been worrying about or putting off dealing with. Yes, you've removed the World's Worst Coping Mechanism – but let's acknowledge that it was nevertheless a coping mechanism and it can take a while for the gap it has left to fill up with wholly positive things. But here's the thing … as exposing as sobriety can be, you've also given yourself the best shot at tackling the tough stuff because you're going to be functioning fully at 100 per cent and not rocking up at a very average 75 per cent or below.

However, if something does go wrong, if you trip up and have a drink, the most important thing is not to give up, accept defeat and resign yourself to going back to the bad old ways for good. Some people (me, for one!) have false starts and it might just take you a few attempts to fully get going. You WILL get there! Remember, if it was easy everyone would be at it. They're not. But you are.

You can use lapses as lessons to power you forward so you have a better idea of how you can navigate the unexpected potholes should they appear again.

Park the guilt, the disappointment, the anxiety and the shame and move on quickly. It's not the end of the world, it's just a bump in the road! Please, please never think you are a failure. You're an absolute badass for even giving this a go. Remind yourself how fabulous you are and don't allow this misfire to make you feel even more shite than you already do.

It's what you decide to do next that's the important thing here – just because you've had a drink today or last night doesn't mean you need to write off the entire weekend, the coming week or the whole month, while you promise yourself you'll start again soon. Start again now. Don't waste any more time on booze. Use the momentum you're gaining and keep flippin' going.

So dust yourself off … and now let's go again!

WHAT TO DO IF YOU HAVE A SETBACK

How you talk to yourself – honestly, but with kindness and compassion – in these moments is key. So here are some important things I want you to consider, whether you've had a wobble or you've fully fallen off the wagon only for it to reverse back over you too.

• First of all, it's REALLY important to acknowledge that taking an extended break from alcohol/ stopping drinking completely is an incredibly difficult thing to do in a society where booze is at every turn. The path to magical and life-changing sobriety is not always going to be easy.

• Go back to your 'why' and your list of things you want to be better in your life (page 73). Remind yourself of where you are trying to get to and resolve to never have your reasons and reminders too far from your mind.

• Take a look at the situation you were in and work out why you had a drink. Was it because you felt like you were missing out? Was it to please others? Do you need to work on developing more coping mechanisms for when life gets tough? Did someone call you 'boring' and you didn't want them to think you were? Did you ignore or fail to recognise a trigger that was bearing down on you like a train?

- Or was it actually something 'simple' – like there was a lack of alcohol-free (AF) options at a bar and you couldn't face drinking yet another Diet Coke or making a fuss? Never be scared of ringing ahead to see what the venue stocks or check out their drinks list online before you go. Forewarned is forearmed!

- Who can you talk to about how you feel? Never hide away feeling like you're on your own because you're absolutely not. Both problematic drinking and glorious sobriety can be lonely places at times, and this is exactly why connection is vitally important. Share with a trusted friend, family member, an online sober buddy or someone who just gets it. Sharing the rough stuff as well as the shiny bits will make you feel so much better and far less alone, I promise you.

- Remind yourself of all the positives that you have enjoyed while you've not been drinking. Consider writing them down so you can see them in black and white. You're waking with a clear head in the mornings, you're far more productive, you've got the 'sober glow' and everyone wants to know your secret, you're saving money, your anxiety levels may well have dropped, you're possibly experiencing a patience you didn't even know you had and on those good days, everything in life seems that little bit brighter. Compare that to how you feel after drinking.

- Take a moment to look at where you are now compared to where you were with your drinking. This might have been your longest dry stint in years. That's brilliant! Don't allow a blip/slip/trip to derail you and keep it in perspective.

- If you're a member of an AF online community, maybe you've not been as active and it's time to get stuck back in. Connections in sobriety are a lifeline and they can be the difference between you staying on track or jumping on the fuck-it button with both feet. Your sober tribe and your fiercest friends will always be there for you. Use them.

- If you've not had much decent sober content in your ears for a while get listening to the Over the Influence (OTI) podcast plus everything else that's out there! Refer back to your quit-lit books that you might have read in your early days and get some sober socials on your daily scroll.

The key thing to do now is to use the situation as a lesson – don't view it as a failure, but an opportunity to add to your sober toolkit. This truly is a chance to use what you now know to arm yourself better for next time.

Now you know what went wrong, let's add to the plan. Complete the following sentence:

Next time I think I might drink, before I do, I am going to:

_____

_____

_____

_____

_____

You're still on the path to becoming a sober superstar. Don't ever give up, and be proud of what you're doing.

CHAPTER 19

The future

Well, this has been quite the journey already! If you are well underway with your 100 days booze-free as you are reading this, then I salute you!

If you are just about to get started then I am excited for all the magic you are about to discover. Yes, it might be hard at times but I hope you now have some ideas for what you need in your alcohol-free (AF) toolkit and you're feeling confident and raring to go.

If you are still feeling sober-curious but hesitating on the edge then that's fine too. I genuinely would love nothing more than for you to bite the bullet, give this a serious go with no ifs or buts and see where it takes you. If in 100 days' time, you decide it's not for you, then *c'est la vie*! But, if in 100 days' time you decide it IS for you ... OMG. The future possibilities are never ending. You know how your life looks with alcohol in it so why not find out how it looks without? You've got nothing to lose and everything to gain.

Just a reminder that you don't need to stand up and declare through a megaphone that you're doing this forever. It is not necessary to commit to never drinking again. Just tell yourself and anyone else who asks that for now, you're not drinking. Once you've broken it down into manageable and digestible chunks, you'll be hurtling towards that triple-figure milestone before you know it and taking huge steps towards shaping a new, unpredictable and exciting AF future for yourself. It doesn't matter where you are in life – be it your age, your circumstances, your finances or your health – it is never (and I cannot stress this enough) too late to change.

I've said a few times in these pages that the simple act of taking alcohol out of the equation can bring benefits and opportunities that never would have occurred to you in your drinking days. So, before I let you go and continue what may well prove to be one of the most magical and life-changing journeys you've ever been on, let's just take a moment to imagine what some of the wider advantages might be for you.

Just a little further down the track, what might future you be enjoying in your new AF life?

CLARITY AND GRATITUDE

The clarity and calmness sobriety brings opens up your capacity to be present and patient with others around you. Whether as a parent, a partner, a friend or a colleague, you're likely to be kinder, to care more, to feel more, to listen harder and to just *be* more for yourself and others. An AF future will actually see you doing the stuff you talked about as a drinker. It's about taking

"The clarity and calmness sobriety brings opens up your capacity to be present and patient with others around you" positive action over taking the empties out, keeping promises instead of forgetting you ever made them and proudly showing up consistently instead of showing yourself up.

Plus, you're going to experience gratitude on another level and you're going to be so very thankful to those who are your biggest sobriety supporters. Thank them and let them know what it means to you as these precious people become part of your journey too.

MAKING MEMORIES

Future you is going to make real memories to last a lifetime because you've taken back control and you're no longer going to let alcohol steal any of them from you.

How many times have you woken up from a night out or a gathering at home trying to piece together the final hours because you've overdone it on the booze and can't for the life of you remember what happened? Or read messages from the group chats and seen social media posts about how it was the 'best night ever' … but for you it feels a bit hazy. It's sort of a waste of a night out if you can't remember anything about it, no?!

At our youngest's christening in 2008, I remember being helped down the stairs of the venue where we were celebrating because, yet again, I'd had (more than) one too many and for some reason I thought it would be a good idea to start on the shots after we'd finished eating. I came home, went to sleep and woke up wondering where everyone had gone and why

"Frustrated feelings of missing out are going to be replaced with the utter glory that is JOMO – the joy of missing out!"

the party had finished. It's embarrassing and of course I regret drinking through key events like this, but that experience has made me even more grateful that being AF now means I get to enjoy the absolute best bits of every celebration with zero regrets and you will too.

The first big gig that I did sober, having been to almost every other show sloshed, was seeing P!nk. Previously, gigs would go something like this for me: drink too much, peak too soon, join a long queue, lose friends, miss best part of gig, go home, wake feeling crap and claim to have had the Best Night Ever.

Sober gigs? Oh lordy. Being completely immersed in the stage show, lights and music. Not missing my favourite songs. Really connecting with the people I am there with. That is SO much better. Seeing Coldplay with my boys was stunning. It literally gave me goosebumps and made me well up. Just sharing the experience with them and being fully present was worth the ticket price alone.

DISCOVERING THE JOMO!

Of course, it's completely normal to feel like you're missing out in the early days of sobriety when you see stuff shared by friends on social media that you've swerved while you get your head around not drinking or that you've not been invited to. Maybe you're also in group chats that ping relentlessly with plans, updates and photos, just to add to your FOMO (fear of missing out). But guess what? Yep, this changes and before you know it those frustrated feelings of missing out are going to be replaced with the utter glory that is JOMO – the joy of missing out!

This is when you really feel the deep benefits of prioritising self-care over self-sabotage; putting yourself first instead of doing your people-pleasing best by saying yes to others; politely but intentionally turning down invites and choosing to do something that makes *you* happy instead; temporarily unplugging from tech and switching off, focusing on the present and feeling grateful for what you have. The list goes on and on. For a while or just every so often, future you is going to find the joy in saying no to others and yes to yourself.

Patience is key and the glimmers of JOMO won't replace the triggers of FOMO overnight. I've already shared with you how my first few Friday nights looked without wine (page 116). Crikey, they were so crap! I was angry, resentful and frothing with FOMO. You will eventually come to realise that once you stop drinking, you're missing out on absolutely nothing and you'll not want to trade the way sobriety makes you feel for anything.

Once you are past your first few milestones and feeling confident, if you want to go to the bar, to the party, to the club (if you have a lot more energy than I do!) then you can. If your social life was brilliant it was just that you struggled with moderation, then that's great. Once you've figured out how to make it work booze-free for you, then get back out there!

But if you find you don't, that actually, you now find the town centre on a Friday night *sort of awful* then that's pretty telling, right? If, once you stop letting booze have a say in how

"Stopping drinking is just the beginning of your future; it's the gateway to huge personal growth" you spend your free time, you find you don't want to be in a crowded, noisy bar, then sobriety will give you the confidence and self-knowledge to be able to say, 'My time is precious and that's not how I want to spend it'. And feel very happy about that decision. You see, JOMO!

CONFIDENCE AND NEW ADVENTURES

Stopping drinking is just the beginning of your future; it's the gateway to huge personal growth. Future you has the potential to achieve so much. Closing the door on alcohol naturally paves the way for so many others to swing open just when you least expect it. It gives you the space you need mentally to consider what you want to achieve and how you start to go about that.

I fell into my forties drunk, hungover and knackered. I excitedly started my fifties feeling calm, content, proud and absolutely buzzing. And I am so proud of myself for every difficult step I took to get there – every drink I turned down, every event I went to feeling apprehensive, every time someone reacted negatively when I said I had stopped drinking. This was *hard* but I did it! And I really can't express the confidence that comes and lights up all areas of your life when you set yourself a challenge like this, put your shoulder to the wheel and just go for it – one step at a time. Future you will feel like you can do anything.

I realised this in 2023. Madonna, who I've adored since I was 12 and seen multiple times live, was set to kick off her world tour in London. However, no one wanted to go with me due to the cost. The tickets alone were a couple of hundred quid. Add to that travel, food and accommodation and it just wasn't happening. However, there wasn't a cat in hell's chance that I was going to miss seeing Madge's Celebration Tour, so I bit the bullet, bought one ticket and went on my own.

Would I have done that as a drinker? Absolutely not. Does not drinking make you brave? Hell yes!

It was an incredible forty-eight hours in the capital. Who knew you could travel by train and not crack the obligatory Train Gin Cans as soon as you depart? Being fully compos mentis and wearing my Big Girl's Pants meant I was able to navigate the Tube all by myself like an actual grown up despite being a nervous northern country bumpkin! I ate out by myself, I talked to people sitting near me in restaurants who were also going to the gig, I took selfies in my seat at the gig wearing my overpriced merch and looking like a radio phone-in competition winner. I even loved the adventure of booking an Airbnb single bedroom in a shared house close to the arena! I took myself off sightseeing the day after as I made my way back to the train station and I couldn't have loved the trip any more if I'd tried. Alcohol would have ruined it. Being sober made it perfect.

Future you is going to say yes to more of the stuff you want to do and if no one wants to do it with you, do it anyway.

"Does not drinking make you brave? Hell yes!"

KNOWING YOURSELF BETTER

Looking back to my fortieth birthday celebrations, just about every single birthday card and gift I received was alcohol themed. Apparently, boozing defined my entire personality. I must have been given at least two dozen bottles of fancy gin, premium flavoured vodka, champagne and Prosecco as gifts as well as toiletries, candles, chocolates and even CHEESE infused with booze. Almost every card had a glass or bottle of booze on the front or wording related to heavy drinking, getting drunk and/or making a dick of yourself while doing so. 'Trust me, you can dance – Vodka', 'I only drink vodka on two occasions – when it's my birthday and when it's not' and 'You know what rhymes with birthday? Vodka.' Hilarious.

As a drinker, how would you describe your personality? What would your friends say about you? Extrovert or introvert? Are you outgoing and socially confident but need fuelling with alcohol to keep you firing on all cylinders and entertaining the masses until you drop? Or perhaps you're a shy and reticent introvert who needs lubricating with a bit of Dutch courage before you go out? Newsflash – a future you without alcohol is going to be a total revelation!

For years, I believed I was the most outgoing person in my social circle and if you were to slice me in two you'd see the word 'extrovert' running through my body like a big stick of Blackpool Rock. Others would describe me as fun and loud and would always encourage me to get the party started – not

...ny encouragement after a few warm-up drinks. I
.. being physically pushed by a friend into the centre of
..pty dance floor at a particularly crap Christmas party and
instructed to get things going on the promise of another drink.

But here's the thing – it turns out I'm not quite the extrovert
I spent the majority of my adult life believing (and being told)
that I was. I'm not socially awkward by any means and I still love
nothing more than a 'reet good do' but I'm no longer interested
in being in the middle of the dance floor and the centre of
attention. I used to declare how I hated being on my own and
that doing anything by yourself is boring. Yep, the opposite of
this is now true.

Future you may well begin to notice shifts in what you
thought were your biggest personality traits. I've seen the shyest
of people who used to drink for courage connect with others
in ways they thought impossible. Drinking alcohol doesn't give
you an ounce of courage; it just gives you a temporary mask to
wear that you can hide behind. If it's something you lean on
heavily, or that your friends associate with you (booze-infused
CHEESE, for God's sake!), then when you take it out of the
equation then it may well take a bit of an adjustment. But aren't
you now excited to get to know yourself a bit better and be able
to always show up as your authentic self?

I can't stand it when people say 'Drinking brings out the
truth ... it shows people exactly who you are!'. Drinking alcohol
changes who we are and it *hides* who we are. It might lessen
inhibitions and temporarily increase confidence but it's fake.

If you want to discover exactly who you are, stopping drinking will allow that to happen.

BEING PART OF A NEW MOVEMENT

Until I found my sober community, every time I tried to give up booze for a while I felt like I was the only one. I wasn't of course, but even in the time since I stopped drinking, things have moved on. The whole wellbeing movement is thriving and the notion of people choosing to live life better without booze is only becoming more popular. As a result of this, the alcohol-free landscape – in terms of what is on offer – has expanded beautifully and is only continuing to grow. Thankfully, the days of a dusty bottle of alcohol-free Kaliber being your only option when you're out are long gone. But not only do you have so much choice when it comes to low and no alcohol drinks at many bars, restaurants and in the supermarket aisles, there are increasingly more opportunities to socialise in venues that are exclusively alcohol-free.

Imagine being somewhere you don't even need to worry if you'll be tempted by booze when you order at the bar because there isn't any, or where you're not looking forward to being the only non-drinker in the place because you'll be surrounded by them. I know, I know … the thought of this right now is probably sending you sideways! I was EXACTLY the same. It's nothing short of brilliant! It's another huge step towards normalising an alcohol-free lifestyle if that's your choice and why shouldn't non-drinkers have somewhere to socialise where they'd rather not be surrounded by booze?

It's definitely a nascent movement at the moment – but the concept of booze-free bars is growing and gaining traction as demand increases. For example, take a look at Karl Considine's social media. The founder of Love From, an inclusive alcohol-free pop-up bar based in Manchester, Karl came on the Over the Influence podcast to tell us about his experience with addiction and how he left his corporate job to pursue Love From. Karl's positive message is that 'cutting out isn't missing out!'. He's right and it really feels like more and more people are looking to socialise alcohol-free.

IAN'S STORY

My 'drinking career' probably started around age sixteen, continuing through my time at university and into my work life. 'Networking', involving drinking, was a big thing in my industry, and this eventually led to me drinking more at home, often alone, as I grew older and more reliant on alcohol, as is the way for so many.

But at some point, I knew it was doing me no good. The law of diminishing returns. Less pleasure, more pain. More anxiety, tiredness, a short fuse, a lack of motivation going towards depression, weight gain, health warnings, worsening hangovers. I wasn't living true to my values and the person I wanted to be.

My dad sadly passed away when I was in my early twenties and my mam didn't fare too well thereafter, albeit she remained with us until only recently, bless her. Let's just say I have seen the fun and the not-so-fun that drinking can bring to relationships and the health of loved ones throughout my life. I had seen how short and unpredictable life can be. I didn't want to waste mine anymore.

In May 2020, as Covid was getting a grip, I thought, *enough is enough*. I had toyed with this before but tried to tackle it alone, white knuckling it until I decided I'd punished myself enough and it really hadn't been that bad in the first place. I discovered the importance of a sober community about four months into a determined stint as I searched online for answers. The Over the Influence podcasts were great – funny, honest and light-hearted. They spoke about what you gained, not what you gave up. I wanted some of this and I've never looked back.

I am now four years alcohol-free. I am over two stone lighter but, more importantly, I feel light-hearted and relaxed. I have got myself fit enough to run some marathons, gained the respect of my family, friends and peers, and I now lead from the front. But do you know what the biggest thing is that I have gained? Self-respect. The people-pleaser has gone and I can now say I like, even love, myself. I'm quietly confident and I know and trust my values. Whatever life throws at my loved ones, I can say hand on heart I show up for them by showing up for myself.

Life can still throw us all curveballs and I won't say it is suddenly amazing. Stopping drinking was really the start of a journey into self-development for me. I now focus on becoming calmer, self-aware, more confident, grateful, fitter, more measured, with clear perspectives and a better work-life balance. No matter what happens from here, I have and will continue to do my best, and I don't see how I will have any regrets. That's important to me, having seen how my parents faired. I hope my children look back on their dad in years

to come and appreciate all he did to show the
values, love, patience and the bravery to do thing
their own way. It would be hard to achieve all of this
if I were still drinking. I struggle to imagine what life
would look like now if I had kept going.

"It's one day, one weekend, one event, one month and one milestone at a time"

CHAPTER 20

. . . .

And finally ...

f I can leave you with just one thing, it is this:

Removing alcohol from your life is not what you *think* you're 'giving up', it's about everything future you is going to gain. Once you realise that you can have a perfectly good time without alcohol, you won't want, or have time, to look back.

How can I say this so confidently without even knowing you? Because I've yet to meet a single person – not ONE – who hasn't experienced the life-changing magic of quitting alcohol since they stopped drinking, regardless of the type of drinker they were. Habitual drinkers, bi-monthly binge drinkers, daily drinkers, occasional drinkers, dependent drinkers and drinkers who described themselves as alcoholic. It doesn't matter how you choose to label your drinking, if at all, or where you put yourself on the vast scale. Choose to remove it, and you're absolutely 100 per cent going to feel better and open yourself up to so many exciting opportunities.

Important reminder – you're not on your own. Refer back to previous chapters in this book and work out exactly how you're going to begin to build your alcohol-free (AF) toolkit in a

way that works best for you. A truly glorious alcohol
is completely in your hands – BUT if the thought ⌣ ⌣ ⌣⌣⌣ a
tad overwhelming right now, you do not need to look too far
ahead. It's one day, one weekend, one event, one month and one
milestone at a time.

I truly believed I'd never stop drinking. Not because I
couldn't stop but because I didn't want to. You are conditioned
from the moment you arrive on this planet to believe and accept
that something that changes your physical and mental state for
the worse is normal and that somehow *you're* the odd one out if
you choose not to. But now I only have one regret in sobriety
and that's not doing it sooner.

Ask yourself, what exactly are you waiting for? Another
decade of frustrated predictability while you're still going round
and round on the boring Hangover Hamster Wheel of Hell? Some
future 'right time' to step into unchartered territory potentially
packed full of fun, opportunity, clarity and excitement? I suggest
you don't wait. The time is now. Future you is going to be so glad
you did this for yourself. It is never too late to rewrite your own
story and change the path of your future.

Part of the life-changing magic you discover in sobriety is
in the ways you'll continue to surprise yourself, from finding
absolute joy in the small things to blowing yourself away in
achieving the brilliantly big things. You're embarking on the
most beautifully bonkers journey of self discovery and at this
stage who knows quite where it will lead! Drinking keeps you
stuck, unable to move forward and grow. Stay on this AF path

and your growth in the future is going to explode. You're going to do things you've never done before and it's all going to start with removing the one thing in your life that you don't even yet realise has been holding you back until now.

Be patient and be kind to yourself at all times. It's unrealistic to promise that removing alcohol fixes everything because it doesn't but what it does do is give you the clarity, space and strength to deal with whatever life throws your way. Believe in magic and trust yourself. Park any preconceived ideas you have about what you *think* not drinking will be like and launch yourself into it with an open mind and a sense of humour. Continuing with old habits will not open new doors and will change nothing about your future.

If you've got a sober itch then scratch it. Curious and intrigued? Jump in. You've got nothing to lose and an absolutely beautiful, colourful and magical whole new world to gain. Do what I did. Try that extended break from booze and just give yourself a chance. You know it's going to be hard but so is drinking. Alcohol will keep you tethered to where you are now, removing it will give you the freedom to fly.

Give yourself the best chance of the most wonderful future because you too deserve to experience the life-changing magic of quitting alcohol. Stop drinking and start living. I promise you, you will not regret it.

Take a big breath, remind yourself why you're doing this, hold your nose and jump in. You won't drown.

Shaz x

"Alcohol will keep you tethered to where you are now, removing it will give you the freedom to fly"

QUIT-LIT

. . . .

If this book has helped you (which I so, so hope it has!) and you want to read more, here are some of my favourites.

The Unexpected Joy Of Being Sober and *Sunshine Warm Sober: The Unexpected Joy of Being Sober – Forever* by Catherine Gray (Aster, 2017 and 2021). You will finish both books smiling, feeling reassured and as though you've just had a big virtual hug from a mate who simply gets it.

Alcohol Explained and *Alcohol Explained 2: Tools for a Stronger Sobriety* by William Porter (Samuel C Watts, 2015 and 2019). These books do what they say on the tin … they explain alcohol – what it does to your mind and body and why so many of us struggle to stop at 'just one'. *Alcohol Explained* was an absolute game changer of a book for me because I finally understood why I was never able to moderate.

The Sober Diaries by Clare Pooley (Hodder and Stoughton, 2017). It's warm, funny and relatable and I just couldn't get enough of it. I felt like Clare was talking about me and to me. I felt connected and as though someone else understood.

This Naked Mind: Control Alcohol, Find Freedom, Discover Happiness & Change Your Life by Annie Grace (Harper Collins, 2018). I didn't find this an easy read (I had to read it twice and REALLY concentrate) as it's quite science heavy, but it will make you ask so many questions about alcohol.

Glorious Rock Bottom by Bryony Gordon (Headline, 2021). It's searingly honest and Bryony takes you on a very personal journey to her rock bottom and then back up to the top again. It's a wonderfully inspiring read from a wonderfully inspiring woman!

Blackout: Remembering The Things I Drank To Forget by Sarah Hepola (Two Roads, 2016). A brutally honest read about the absolute lows of Sarah's alcohol addiction. Funny, warm and another inspiring story!

Alcohol Lied To Me by Craig Beck (Viral Success Limited, 2010). A really good read.

MILESTONES TRACKER

I wrote earlier about how important it is to look forward to and celebrate your milestones. As we have said many times now in these pages, what you are doing is HARD and you deserve to take a moment to reflect on all the difficult moments and congratulate yourself for getting through them. It's so helpful to keep a record of your sober journey. You can do it through voicenotes, videos, social media posts, however you want, really. Here are a few things to consider at each important stage – one week, two weeks, one month, fifty days, seventy-five days and one hundred days:

- How are you feeling today?
- What changes have you noticed since you passed your last milestone?
- How much money have you saved by not spending it on booze?
- Highlight something you've done alcohol-free that you didn't think possible.
- What are you grateful for today?
- What are you most proud of in your alcohol-free journey so far?